A Good Night's Sleep

Addressing Insomnia, Stress and Digital Toxicity

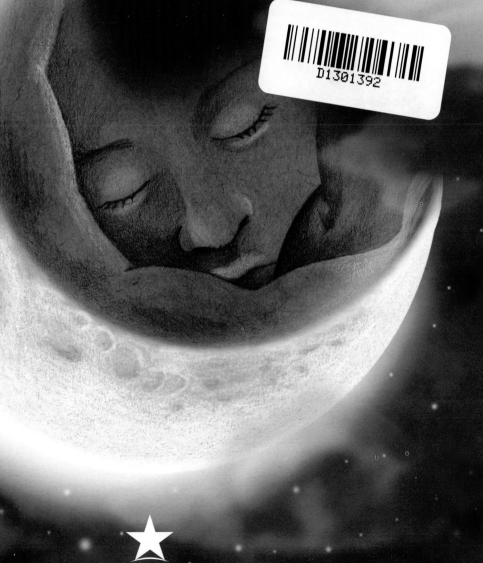

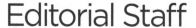

Editorial Staff

Author: Brian Luke Seaward, PhD

Executive Editor: Ryan Picarella, MS, SPHR

Managing Editor: Brittanie Leffelman, MS

Contributing Editor: Carie Maguire

Design/Illustration: Adam Paige

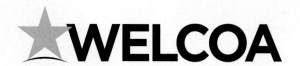

17002 Marcy Street, Suite 140 | Omaha, NE 68118
PH: 402-827-3590 | FX: 402-827-3594 | welcoa.org

Table of Contents

About **WELCOA**

The Wellness Council of America (WELCOA) was established as a national not-for-profit organization in the mid 1980s through the efforts of a number of forward-thinking business and health leaders. Drawing on the vision originally set forth by William Kizer, Sr., Chairman Emeritus of Central States Indemnity, and WELCOA founding Directors that included Dr. Louis Sullivan, former Secretary of Health and Human Services, and Warren Buffett, Chairman of Berkshire Hathaway, WELCOA has helped influence the face of workplace wellness in the U.S.

Today, WELCOA has become one of the most respected resources for workplace wellness in America. With a membership in excess of 5,000 organizations, WELCOA is dedicated to improving the health and well-being of all working Americans. Located in America's heartland, WELCOA makes its national headquarters in one of America's healthiest business communities—Omaha, Nebraska.

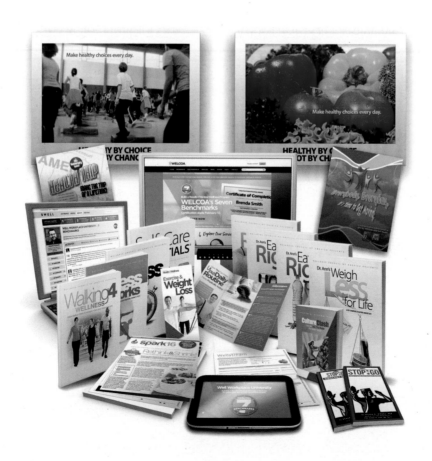

About **Brian Luke Seaward, PhD**

Brian Luke Seaward is regarded as one of the foremost experts in the field of stress management and a pioneer in the field of mind-body-spirit healing. He has authored more than twelve books, including the classic best sellers, *Stand Like Mountain, Flow Like Water, The Art of Calm* and *Stressed Is Desserts Spelled Backward*. As a TEDx speaker, the wisdom of Brian Luke Seaward can be found quoted in PBS specials, The Chicago Tribune, The Huffington Post, college graduation speeches, medical seminars, boardroom meetings, church sermons, and keynote addresses all over the world. He is respected throughout the international community as an accomplished teacher, consultant, motivational speaker, author, visionary, and mentor. His corporate clients include Hewlett Packard, Wells Fargo, Procter & Gamble, Conoco Oil, Motorola, Quaker Oats, John Deere, BP-Amoco, Blue Cross/Blue Shield, Maxtor-Seagate, Organic Valley Dairy, U.S. Army, and many others. Former Good Morning America host, Joan Lunden says, "Dr. Seaward's words have touched my life profoundly and helped me to find grace and dignity, the patience and compassion needed to navigate my ever-changing course. They have helped me understand that it is the way I choose to see the world that I will create the world I see." He currently serves on the faculty of The Graduate Institute in Bethany, CT and is the Executive Director of the Paramount Wellness Institute in Boulder, CO. He can be reached via his website, **www.brianlukeseaward.net**.

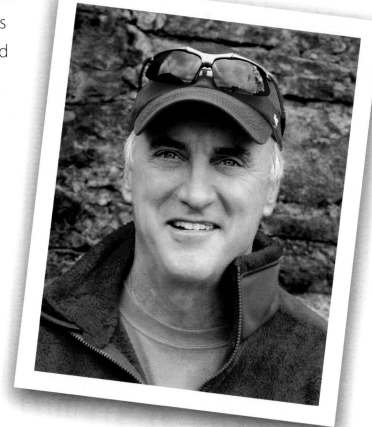

FOREWORD

Sleep: Nature's Medicine

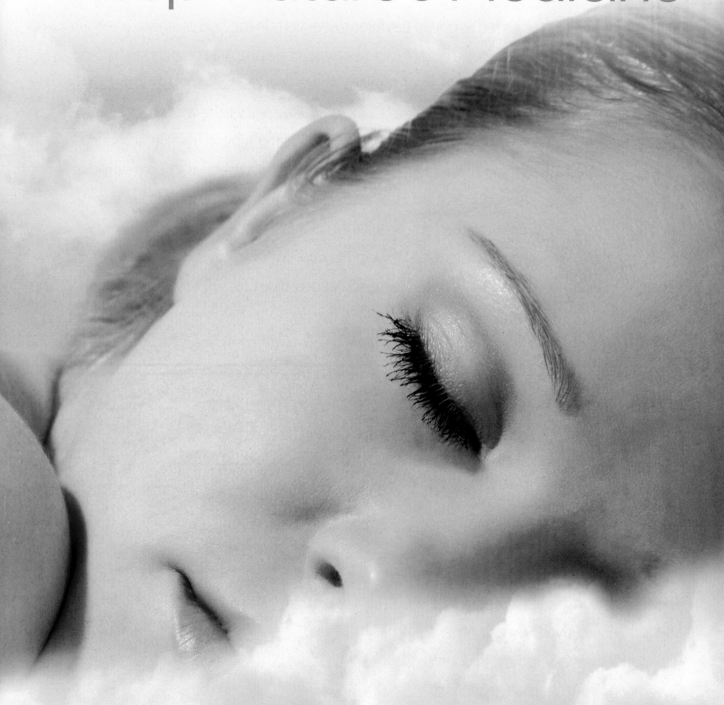

We spend on average one-third of our entire lives sleeping. For most people that equates to 26 years of sleep—or at least 26 years spent *trying* to sleep. Sleep is one of the few areas in health and wellness that all experts agree on. Health and wellness professionals not only concur that sleep is incredibly important and most of us don't get enough, but they have begun to incorporate sleep resources and education into well-rounded wellness program offerings. This book is a comprehensive resource for educating us about the benefits of sleep and arming us with strategies for sleeping better and improving our overall well-being.

What makes *A Good Night's Sleep,* by Dr. Brian Luke Seaward, a truly special book is that it explores factors that affect our sleep that most people haven't thought about yet—factors that are absolutely within our control that we can start improving today. Implementing the ideas in this book can help you combat insomnia and the devastating impact it can have on our lives, our jobs and those around us. Through research, stories, activities and practical tips, Dr. Seaward takes us on a journey to discover how we can all rest easier. We live in a brave new world full of incredible technology, and while it has improved many aspects of our lives, it can rob us of our sleep and ultimately our health. Learn tools, tricks and practices to set healthy boundaries and ensure that you get a good night's sleep every night. When it comes to the quantity and quality of our sleep, we simply cannot do more with less. Sleep is truly nature's medicine.

Cheers,

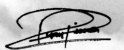

Ryan Picarella
President
WELCOA

About Ryan Picarella

As WELCOA's President, Ryan brings immense knowledge and insight from his career that spans over a decade in the health and wellness industry. He is a national speaker, healthcare consultant, and has designed and executed award winning wellness programs. Known for his innovative and pragmatic approach to workplace wellness, Ryan looks forward to furthering the WELCOA mission and vision and continuing to position the organization for success for the future.

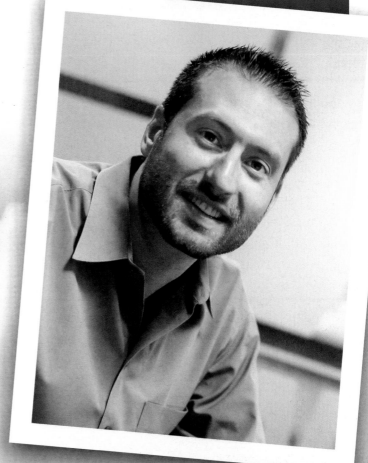

INTRODUCTION

Counting Sheep

Back in 2005, I was invited to give a wellness presentation to a group of software engineers on the topic of stress and insomnia. The presentation, *A Good Night's Sleep,* was part of an ongoing wellness series, but unlike other topics, this one struck a loud chord. The room was packed; in fact, standing room only. While the wellness director was ecstatic at the turnout (her best ever for a wellness event) the implications of the topic's popularity were disconcerting, both to her and me.

Under the premise of full disclosure, I sleep really well. In fact, throughout my whole life, the dream-weaver has been very good to me. I sleep like a log—every night. It might be my regular exercise routine. It might be my meditation practice, a healthy diet, or perhaps it's just plain luck. Regardless of my sleep habits, in terms of insomnia, I had much to learn and hit the ground running with this topic. What I have learned is not comforting. I knew that stress played a role in insomnia, but I had no idea just how significant a role it was. Perhaps as no surprise to you who are reading this book, the association between stress and insomnia is colossal.

In the preparation for that worksite wellness talk on insomnia (and several others since), I did a lot of research. I was flabbergasted to learn how prevalent a problem poor sleep quality is in America. As part of my research, I sat down and interviewed a nationally renowned sleep expert for over four hours. I learned a lot. His take on America's insomnia epidemic was not promising. Several comments he made sent a chill up my spine, including this: "Sleep medications are way over prescribed by the medical community. In the U.S., we treat the symptoms, not the cause." He also said that the brain has over 300 neuropeptides (perhaps many more yet undiscovered) associated with cognition and optimal brain function. Many, if not all of these, are affected by the foods we eat, or nutrients we don't consume. Medical science has three (out of 300) brain chemicals well researched: serotonin (the happy hormone), dopamine (the pleasure hormone) and epinephrine (a catecholamine associated with stress). "To be honest, in terms of depression, insomnia, and other brain-related matters, we are quite embryonic in our understanding of what we are doing with neuropharmaceuticals and brain chemistry," he concluded.

He made some recommendations which I in turn, would like to share:

> "Many books on the topic of health end with the phrase: Check with your physician before… I would say, find/select a physician who understands the mind-body-spirit connection and supports integrative medicine (e.g., acupuncture, nutrition, craniosacral therapy, etc.). Any doctor whose first course of action is to prescribe medications is a red flag. If this is the case, find another physician. A medical prescription should be the last course of action, not the first. Also, find a physician who has a solid background in nutrition. So much of optimal brain chemistry begins with proper nutrition."

In 2009, on the savvy suggestion of Dr. David Hunnicutt, my presentation, *A Good Night's Sleep,* became a WELCOA webinar. David called me the first day it aired to tell me that it had over 11,000 hits. Once again a chord was struck. In turn, that webinar sowed the seeds for this book in the WELCOA Workplace Wellness Series, one that both he and WELCOA's President Ryan Picarella strongly support. Like other books in this series, this book attempts to provide an overview of a very complex, yet compelling topic. As such, I simply can't address all the aspects of this topic in this book in great detail (each chapter could be a book itself), but it's a start. And after learning of the profound connection between screen technology and insomnia, I felt this merited its own chapter as well. The topics, sleep, insomnia, stress, digital toxicity and mindfulness are all related (and you will see both an overlap and repetition in this content throughout this book—as the expression goes, review never hurts). We invite you to use this book as a stepping-stone for further exploration in this very important aspect of wellness. Here is wishing all of you a good night's sleep, always.

Best wishes, sweet dreams and inner peace.

Brian Luke Seaward, PhD

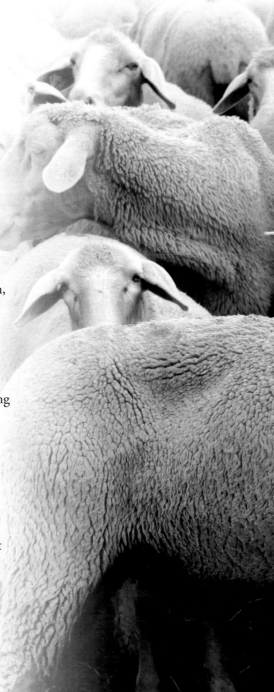

CHAPTER ONE

America: A Sleep-Deprived Nation

*Early to bed and early to rise, makes
a man healthy, wealthy and wise.*

BEN FRANKLIN

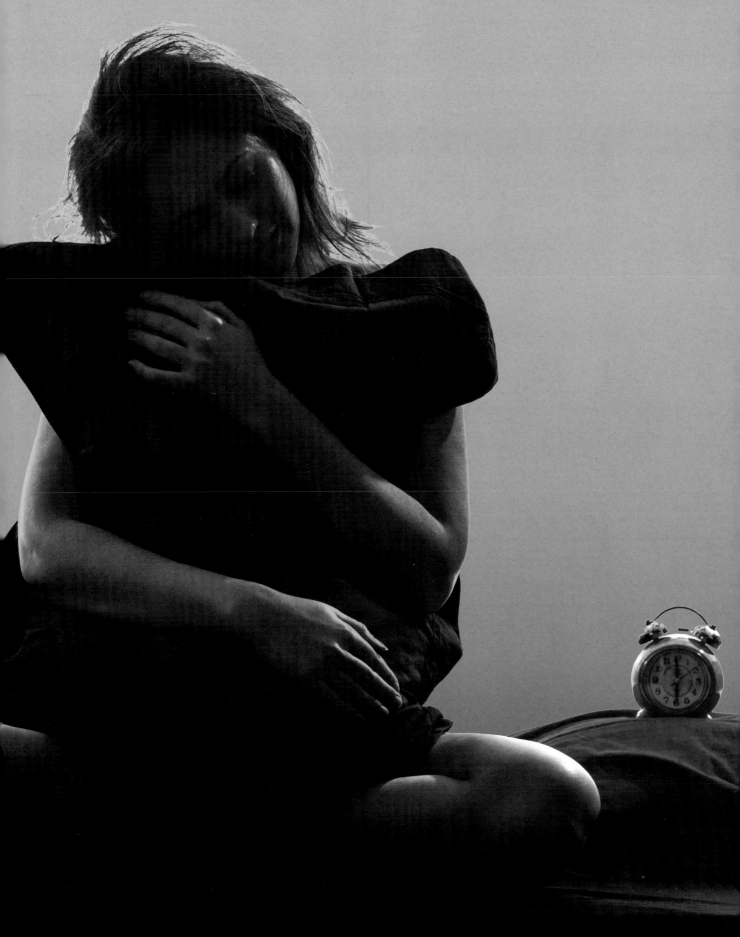

CHAPTER ONE

America: A Sleep-Deprived Nation

Sara doesn't sleep well at night, and she hasn't for years. Over a cup of coffee she confides in me that it takes hours for her to fall asleep, only to wake up several times in the course of the night, staring at the alarm clock, wishing it were morning. Sara is not alone in her quest for a good night's sleep. She has joined the ranks of millions of restless Americans who claim a similar disturbance in what should be a most pleasurable experience; one that we spend one-third of our lives engaged in. The rebound effect of poor quality sleep reveals itself in the normal waking hours through poor work productivity, irritability, anxiety, poor communication skills, slow reaction time when driving, questionable parenting skills and several behaviors that are less than becoming of one's optimal potential. America's dependence on coffee is as much a symptom as a possible cause of the problem.

America is a sleep-deprived nation! According to a recent survey by the National Sleep Foundation, over 60% of Americans suffer from poor sleep quality resulting in everything from falling asleep on the job and absenteeism to marital problems, chronic health issues and car accidents. Moreover, our growing obsession with screen-held devices now plays a leading role in this as well; the newest science reveals that both screen light and WiFi microwaves affect our biological clocks, and not in a good way.

A quick check of the nation's pulse reveals that insomnia, in all its many forms, has become one more aspect on a growing list of national health epidemics. Moreover, insomnia is now linked to many chronic diseases, from coronary heart disease to cancer. The newest evidence links insomnia to obesity. The lack of a good night's sleep, as a common health issue, is made quite evident with the proliferation of pharmaceutical television ads promising an insomnia cure to the newest health epidemic of the high-tech age. It's no secret that sleep medications are among those at the top of the list for prescriptions in the U.S.

Perhaps most troublesome is the dramatic incidence of insomnia reported in middle school and high school students whose brains are still developing. For adults and children alike, a succession of restless nights becomes a battle of thought processes between the conscious mind's inability to turn off, and the unconscious mind's inability to communicate essential information through dreams. The end result is that both sides claim casualties, and neither side is victorious. America, as a sleep-deprived nation, also gives a whole new meaning to the expression "the coming zombie apocalypse." Many would say it's already here.

In our rapidly changing world where it is typical for the average person to become allured by the bombardment of screen time sensory stimulation, it has become quite common for people to shave off precious time on either

60% of Americans suffer from poor sleep quality resulting in everything from falling asleep on the job and absenteeism to marital problems, chronic health issues and car accidents.

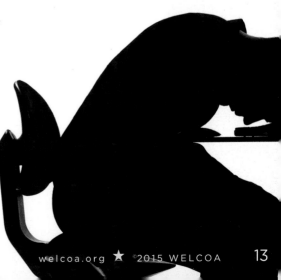

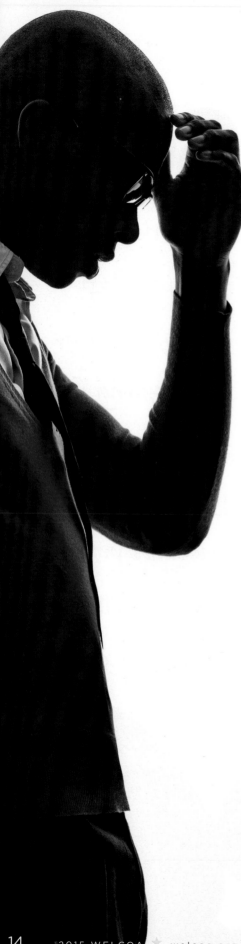

end of one's allocated nocturnal sleep allotment. The end result is that we sacrifice our long-term health for short-term pleasure. Oddly enough, many of the Millennial Generation and Generation X'ers feel that sleep is a form of surrender; surrender in avoiding responsibilities, surrender to curiosity (Internet surfing) or merely surrender to exhaustion. By and large, people hate to give in to surrender, as it conveys a sense of weakness. For some, (perhaps many) people who see hyper-productivity as a badge of honor, eight hours of sleep is perceived as a weakness compared to the now common four or five hours. Ironically, the lack of consistently good sleep habits can become a serious lifelong weakness where one's personal health is the biggest casualty. Simply stated, for those who hold fast to today's 24/7 behaviors that negate a good night's sleep, prolonged health and wellness are inadvertently sabotaged. Many compromise a good night's sleep for a mediocre day at the office, all the while searching for happiness. What's the answer? To paraphrase a famous quote: "Sleep is bliss, follow your bliss."

Americans may be sleep deprived, but it doesn't have to be this way. There are simple solutions and positive behaviors that can bring healthy sleep habits back into balance. To begin with, a solid awareness of the problem is the first step to resolving it. The bottom line is this: Quality sleep is essential to your optimal health.

Insomnia Defined

Insomnia is a term used to define the inability to get a good night's sleep. Recently, it has become a catch-all phrase to describe a multitude of sleep-related problems. So pervasive is insomnia, some physicians now call it a "Wakefulness Disorder." Neither a disease nor a syndrome, insomnia can best be defined as a symptom of other health related issues, from sleep apnea (irregular breathing), depression, chronic pain and acid reflux to emotional stress. Insomnia is often characterized as the inability to fall asleep, stay asleep or repeatedly waking up. The disruption of "sound sleep" is often suggestive of other health concerns or issues (e.g., menopause, side effects of prescriptions, or psychological problems such as stress, anxiety, or depression).

The Purpose of Sleep

In any given day there are 24 hours. In an ideal world (no matter where you live on the planet), eight of these hours each day are deemed necessary for sleep, so that one can function optimally during the remaining 16 hours. When you do the math, the numbers don't lie. We spend about one-third of our lives sleeping. Given this amount of time, one might conclude that quality sleep is not only important, but essential to one's health and well-being. This is true. Death and taxes may be a certainty in life, but to this list we can add sleep, for without adequate sleep, the waking hours can be a living hell.

It is interesting to note that back in the early '70s several DJ's across the country would seek a greater share of their potential target audience by pulling on-air publicity stunts. One such promotional gimmick included staying on the air for days on end with barely more than a few bathroom breaks. In what sounds like one more urban legend tall tale, each DJ who tried this foolish challenge began to show signs of psychosis within 36-48 hours of sleep deprivation. In essence, without adequate sleep, they became totally incoherent and unable to perform their job. This practice of marathon DJ'ing abruptly stopped when the end result proved to be embarrassing, if not disastrous for the listening public. Remarkably, each sleep-deprived DJ recovered fully once sleep was reintroduced into their routine. Identical psychotic behavior was also observed with the finalists of marathon dances and promotional free car giveaway contests (remember the advertising phrase: "Put your hands on a Toyota and never let go?"). From this absurd data collection of case studies, it was concluded that not only is sleep each night important, but essential to our mental and physical health. Least we forget that to this day, sleep deprivation is a form of torture in many countries around the world.

The Study of Sleep

The subject of sleep as a topic of scientific investigation began, in earnest, about 50 years ago, after World War II. For most of this period scientists were at a loss to explain the exact importance of sleep, other than in general terms; rest and rejuvenation. It was also at this time that rapid eye movement (REM) was first fully noted, but not clearly understood. Interestingly, most of the sleep research centered on what happens to us mentally and physically when we don't sleep.

Why do we need to sleep? Rest and rejuvenation may seem like the most intuitive (and obvious) answers, but the mind-body-spirit dynamic is far more complex than this. Anyone who ever tried to pull an all-nighter in college quickly realized that the attempted gains were short lived, and that both mind and body can only be pushed so far before both memory and physical stamina give out. Originally, one theory suggested that sleep was thought to be a way to avoid dangerous nocturnal, carnivorous predators. As sleep research began in earnest, physiology experts cited "restoration," where the metabolic activity of cells works to repair tissue damage and keep our bodies in homeostasis, as one of the primary reasons for sleep. Psychologists, in turn, explain that the conscious mind needs to rest so that the unconscious mind can problem solve and consolidate memories. Dreams (whether you remember them or not) are the mind's way of resolving personal issues, and offering solutions to problems begging for attention. Dreams help us navigate our next day journey, when we take the time to decipher them.

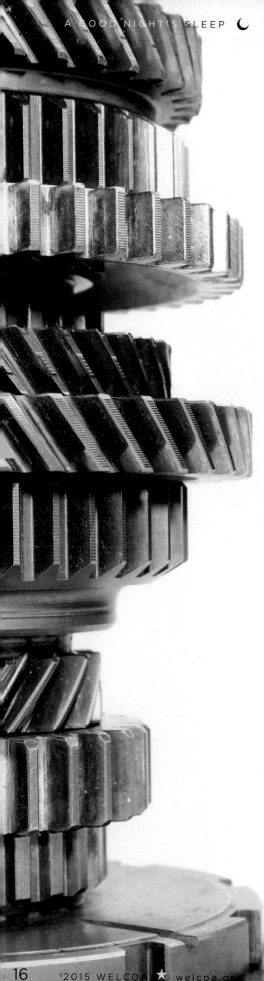

With the introduction of electroencephalogy (EEG), a way to measure brain waves, it was revealed that as one goes from a conscious state (awake) to an unconscious state (sleep), the amplitude (spike) of brain wave activity decreases significantly. As such, researchers presumed that the brain, like a muscle, slows down its activity dramatically. This turned out not to be the case. In the past decade, via the use of advances in technology, sleep research has become a lot more complex and comprehensive. With the use of brain scans, brain imaging and MRI's, medical science has looked deeply into the brain to understand its secrets; several of which have been revealed regarding the science of sleep. Here is what they have found:

The brain doesn't turn off when we fall asleep. Rather a whole different set of brain cells (glial cells) are busy at work washing over the brain in a synchronized flow, cleansing brain tissue of "toxic amyloid proteins" which are now known to cause problems (e.g., dementia, Alzheimer's) if amounts accumulate over time. Brain physiologists refer to these toxins as "brain garbage." Simply stated, the trash has to be removed nightly across the sensitive and protective blood-brain barrier for optional cognitive abilities.

Brain cells in mice that are not allowed to rest show signs of collapse. The same is thought to be true for humans.

Brain cells that fire repeatedly, without rest, are observed to create free radicals (which can then destroy cell membranes, RNA, DNA and mitochondria, accelerating the aging process). During sleep, brain neurons create antioxidants that destroy free radicals.

Additionally, here are some other reasons for sleep:

Sleep may help maintain the integrity of telomeres (the ends of the DNA strand involved with cell duplication). Hence, sleep delays the aging process (giving a whole new meaning to the expression "beauty rest.")

Sleep helps regulate cell metabolism and body weight.

Growth hormone is active during sleep to help regulate the repair of damaged tissue (from exercise or injury).

During sleep, energy from metabolic activity is devoted to repair of bone and muscle tissues.

With the use of brain scans, brain imaging and MRI's, medical science has looked deeply into the brain to understand its secrets; several of which have been revealed regarding the science of sleep.

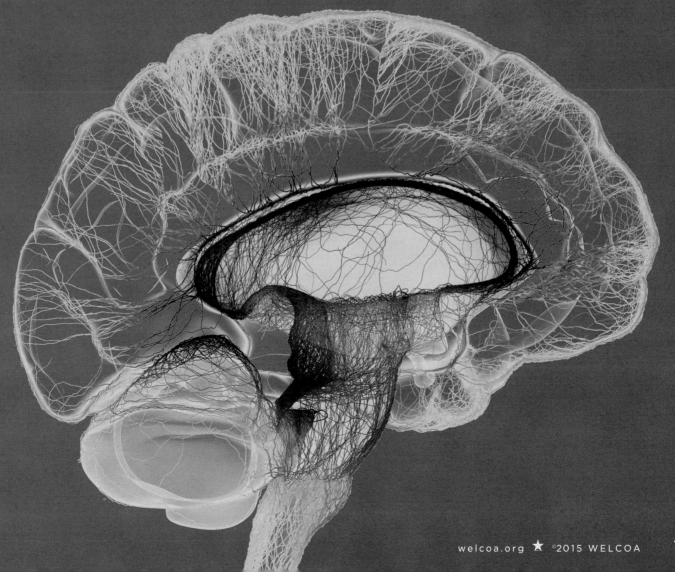

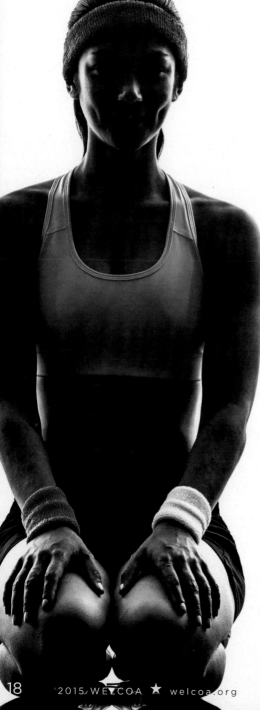

Cardiovascular exercise ensures proper blood flow to all the body's tissues, including the brain.

The Causes of Insomnia

In the past 50 years of sleep research, what has become very obvious is the multitude of reasons why people don't sleep well. As you read this list, keep in mind that with the exception of stress, each of these factors only contributes a small fraction to the total problem of insomnia, or what is now being called "Wakefulness Disorder." Stress is attributed to well over half of the reasons why people claim not to sleep well or lay awake at night eluding a good night's sleep altogether (this topic will be discussed in the next chapter).

☽ **Lack of Exercise:** The human body was designed to be active. Today most people are quite sedentary, meaning they are very, very inactive. Inactivity is often associated with chronic physical disabilities prevalent with the elderly. Today, the young and old alike are quite sedentary, more so now than ever before. The body may like rest, but it also craves exercise. Cardiovascular exercise ensures proper blood flow to all the body's tissues, including the brain. The effects of inactivity on the body are quite profound and often resemble those of the aged population. In no uncertain terms, inactivity accelerates the aging process. Exercise may not be the fountain of youth, but it definitely promotes a good night's sleep.

☽ **Shift Work:** People who work during the evening and early morning hours throw off their internal body clock. Chronobiology is the study of the body's circadian rhythms, regulated by sunlight. In turn, circadian rhythms regulate everything from hormone secretion to a host of metabolic activities. When the human body's circadian rhythms are finely tuned, optimal health prevails. Late night shift work fights the body's natural tendencies to sleep during the hours of darkness. While some people may adapt to this time change, others notice the long-term negative effects on their health, starting with poor sleep habits during the daylight hours, particularly when other family members sleep during the normally accepted time period of darkness.

☽ **Frequent Urination:** There are several reasons why people need to empty their bladder in the middle of the night, including bladder size, pregnancy, the side effects of prescriptions (such as hypertension medications) and men who have issues with their prostate. As anyone can tell you, it is hard to sleep with a full bladder, and for many, it's hard to fall back asleep in the middle of the night after a trip to the bathroom.

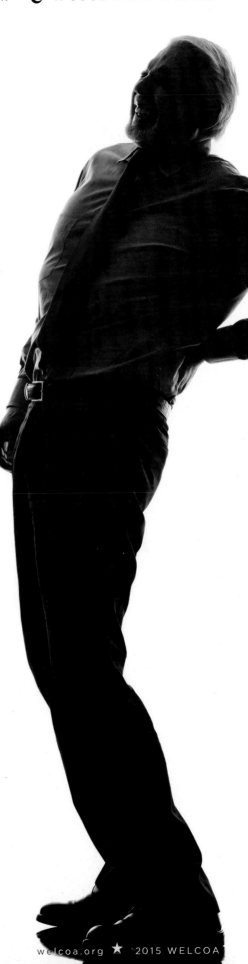

☾ **Chronic Pain:** Joint pain, muscle pain, angina, skin irritations and other types of neurological conditions are just a few examples of chronic pain. When the mind is preoccupied with pain and discomfort, the ability to fall asleep and stay asleep is often compromised. Chronic pain as a symptom of chronic disease, such as fibromyalgia, rheumatoid arthritis and even Lyme disease compromise the conscious mind's ability to turn off and rest.

☾ **Medications:** The average American is on several medications, each with side effects and many with complicating interactions, including frequent urination, anxiety, muscle cramps, muscle tension, headaches and many more, all of which can interrupt a good night's sleep.

☾ **Sleep Apnea:** Sleep apnea is a condition where one's ability to breathe comfortably during the night is compromised by frequent pauses (apnea). There are two types of sleep apnea: 1) obstructive and 2) central. Either type denies adequate oxygen to the brain (and other parts of the body). The consequences can be quite serious, even deadly (see Appendix A: FAQs About Insomnia, Stress and Wellness, #5).

☾ **Jet Lag:** Our body's physiology is designed to function well at the speed of life, which up until jet airplanes was pretty much living in one time zone. The advent of jet propulsion technology changed all of this. While one can travel with great ease halfway around the world in several hours, the toll on the body's biological clock (also known as circadian rhythms) is quite noticeable, particularly when you fly east, in the direction of the planet's rotation. Even traveling one time zone can throw off our circadian rhythms (and the same thing happens each Spring and Fall with the switch to/from daylight savings time).

☾ **Cell Phone Use:** Cell phones may provide great freedom and convenience, but there is a hidden (and dangerous) cost to a wireless connection. Cell phones give off low levels of microwave radiation (known in the field of physics as Extremely Low Frequency (ELF) vibrations). Through the process of sympathetic resonance, brain cells that entrain to these vibrations can mutate into cancerous cells. Additionally, ELFs from cell phones held close to the head are also known to affect the pineal gland's ability to make melatonin, thus affecting sleep patterns.

> A recent Harvard study by Dr. Charles Czeisler found that the artificial blue light emitted from various electronic devices arouses brain neurons throwing off circadian rhythms including the sleep hormone, melatonin.

Cordless phones are no safer, as they too operate on a wireless signal. According to a recent Huffington Post article, 63% of people ages 18-29 bring their phones to bed with them. Cell phones are also noted to sabotage people's sex life.

☾ **Screen Addictions:** Have you ever noticed that people have their eyes glued to the screens of their tablets, smart phones or laptops at all hours of the day and night? People who exhibit this type of behavior are noted as being hypervigilant, a characteristic noted in people who have PTSD. The use of technology is wonderful, but it does have some drawbacks. One such concern is the light emitted from these screen devices that causes a hormonal shift in brain chemistry, known as melatonin suppression. A recent Harvard study by Dr. Charles Czeisler found that the artificial blue light emitted from various electronic devices arouses brain neurons throwing off circadian rhythms including the sleep hormone, melatonin. Keep in mind that airplane mode is still a WiFi signal.

☾ **Stress:** Stress, specifically, emotional stress in the form of anxiety, worry, resentment and frustration lets the mind run wild with thoughts and emotions that keep the conscious mind awake. Research shows that over 50% of insomnia cases are the result of stress. The majority of people who claim not to sleep very well also confide that they have a very active mind that they cannot shut off when their head hits the pillow. (The next two chapters will highlight many aspects of stress.)

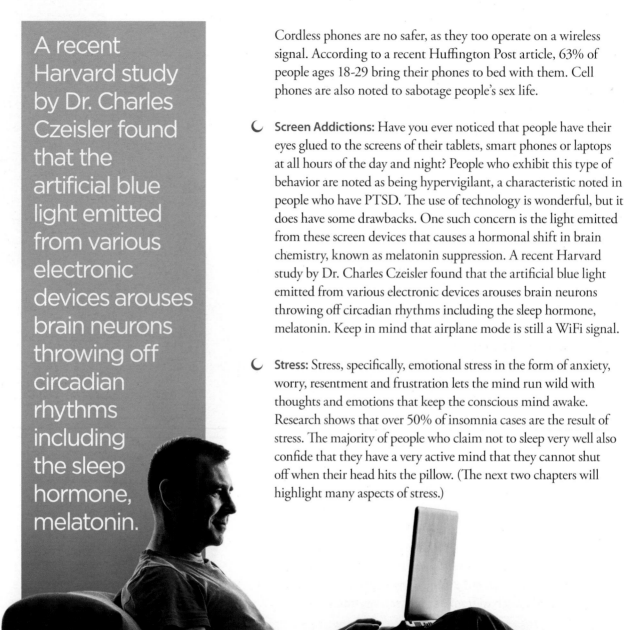

The Effects of Insomnia

What happens when you don't get enough sleep each night? The list of effects from poor sleep read like a script from the popular TV show, *The Walking Dead:*

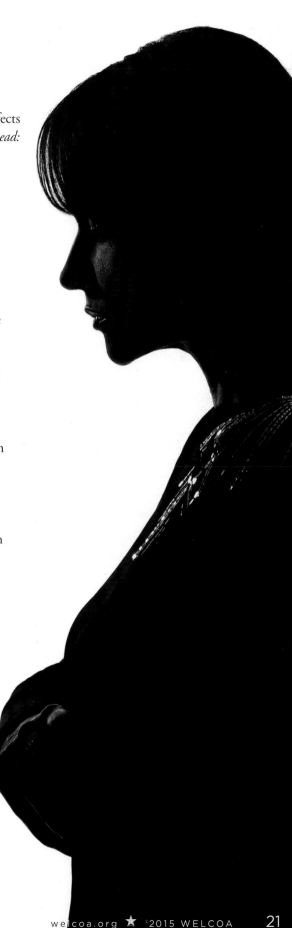

☾ **A Depressed Immune System:** Perhaps the most significant casualty of disruptive sleep patterns is a compromised immune system. Research reveals that sleep is essential for a highly functioning immune system. When sleep cycles are interrupted, the family of white blood cells decreases, hence the immune system is greatly compromised leading the way to a host of health-related problems.

☾ **Lapse of Attention:** Attention spans are short to begin with these days, but lack of sleep makes them even shorter. Not being able to gather information also compromises our ability to process and remember it. A lack of sleep is analogous to a cell phone that needs its battery charged, or when cell phone calls keep getting dropped due to a poor connection.

☾ **Slow Thinking:** The speed at which the brain processes information is nothing short of amazing. This speed and efficacy is greatly compromised when sleep is restricted or denied altogether. Slow thinking decreases one's reaction time, which is not crucial when surfing the Internet, but very critical when driving or operating machines at work. It's also crucial when having a conversation with colleagues, friends or family members. Slow thinking also means poor judgment skills, whether it's attending a staff meeting or driving a car.

☾ **Irritability:** People who sleep poorly are more likely to react than respond, when stressed. They also take things more personally and reveal a quick temper with a shorter fuse. In essence, people become on edge, and stay on edge all day long.

☾ **Poor Memory:** Healthy brain cells are the gateway to a good memory. The current theory suggests that during sleep, the brain sorts out important information and tosses the rest. Poor sleep quality inhibits the sorting process, making memory retrieval all the more difficult in the waking hours.

☾ **Anxiety and Depression:** There is a HUGE correlation between depression and insomnia, with several chicken and egg

SLEEPLESS IN AMERICA

The National Geographic Society is renowned for its documentaries about nature, wildlife and remote world cultures, but in December of 2014 they came out with a stunning documentary titled, Sleepless in America. The take-home message: Americans are exhausted, sleep is elusive to many Americans and chronic sleep deprivation may have irreparable damage to one's health. According to their estimates, 40% of American adults are sleep deprived and 70% of adolescents are far short of the proverbial eight hours of sleep each night. The association between an over-stimulated America (e.g., smart phones and video games) and a sleep-deprived America was not lost on the experts interviewed in this film. Moreover, whereas weekends were once a time to regain some work-life balance (e.g., afternoon naps), people today are so overworked that they not only miss their nap time, but tend to stay up late on weekends as well.

Citing the most current research, experts revealed that not only are poor sleep habits associated with cancer, heart disease, diabetes and several other diseases, but those who are chronically sleep deprived tend to have an increased appetite (for fatty foods). People who miss the suggested eight hours of sleep tend to eat 500 more calories per day than those who do get a good night's sleep. The take-home message the producers of this movie want viewers to remember: sleep inspires creativity, re-balances one's emotions, helps refresh cardiovascular health, metabolic health and gives a great boost to the immune system.

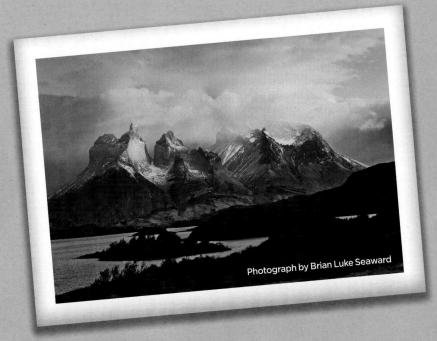

Photograph by Brian Luke Seaward

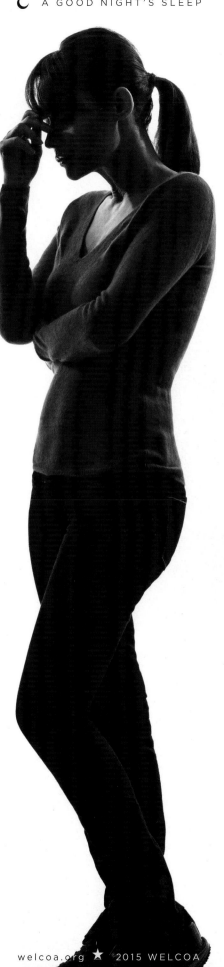

comparisons (i.e., which causes which). Regardless, anxiety and depression may inhibit a good night's sleep, but insomnia seems to worsen each of these mental conditions, forming what is called a "negative feedback loop." (This is addressed in more detail in Chapter 4.).

☾ **Decrease in Work Productivity:** The eight hours we sleep each night is an investment in the quality of work in our waking hours. Poor sleep equals poor work quality. In a recent *TIME* magazine article, titled *The Power of Sleep,* it was stated that 40% of adults admitted to falling asleep at work. And that is when they actually come to work. Insomnia is one of the leading reasons why people call in sick. To a stressed worker, absenteeism often feels justified because the boundary between work and home has become non-existent with 24 hour access via emails, texting, phone calls and other means of social media.

Insomnia and Work Productivity

Insomnia is not only a personal health issue; it's a corporate wellness issue. Behaviors associated with a sleep-deprived culture easily bleed into a dysfunctional workforce. Having a cognitive deficit at work shows up in the following ways:

☾ **Absenteeism:** Insomnia is one of the primary reasons people call in sick.

☾ **Presenteeism:** Presenteeism is a word to describe people who show up to work, but don't do anything when they are there. Poor sleep habits are a leading cause of presenteeism.

☾ **Lack of Focus:** Concentration skills are greatly compromised at work when workers are suffering from sleep deprivation. Lack of focus impedes work quality.

☾ **Mistakes and Accidents:** According to the National Safety Council, 95% of worksite accidents and Inspection Failure Rate (IFR) are the result of human error (where the mind was elsewhere, also known as not being present). Mental fatigue, poor concentration skills and poor reaction time are all part of this accident equation.

☾ **Interpersonal Difficulties:** When several people are put together under the roof of one workspace, personality conflicts are sure

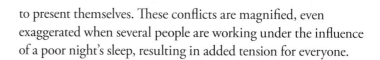

to present themselves. These conflicts are magnified, even exaggerated when several people are working under the influence of a poor night's sleep, resulting in added tension for everyone.

☾ **Poor Work Attitude:** Members of EAP programs, Human Resources and wellness programs support the claim that people with sleep disorders are more likely to manifest a poor work attitude, which like a virus, can spread to others within the work environment, and infect nearly everyone, making for a toxic work environment.

Stress and Insomnia

Question: What keeps people up at night, wide awake while others are fast asleep? Answer: A troubled mind.

When some aspect of ourselves (usually the ego) feels threatened, the mind (and the brain which houses the mind) quickly becomes engaged in the stress response. Thoughts, in the way of neural impulses, ricochet all over the brain's interior, like a busy intersection during rush hour. Images of brain waves of people engaged in these thought processes look anything but tranquil. When people are questioned as to what events and aspects of their lives can cause so much stress that they cannot sleep, the list of stressors is endless, yet the commonalities of these problems are very familiar as noted in the list below:

- ❯ Work responsibilities
- ❯ Finances/personal debt issues
- ❯ Job security/dead-end job
- ❯ Marital issues
- ❯ Family issues
- ❯ Health care issues
- ❯ Childcare issues
- ❯ Raising teenagers issues
- ❯ Eldercare issues
- ❯ Career/purpose in life issues
- ❯ Retirement issues
- ❯ Other personal issues

As Above, So Below

Do our inner thoughts mirror the world we live in? While it's true that our world today is quite complex, and perhaps much more stressful, certainly more busy, than generations ago, there are time tested ways to find the calm (and remain calm) in the storm of our 24/7 on-demand, social networking, fast-paced culture. Good sleep management is a combination of good stress management, good time management and good healthy boundaries. The expression, "As Above, So Below," refers to the timeless wisdom that reminds us to return to the center of tranquility, that which we are a part of that connects us to the whole. Before we examine ways to promote a good night's sleep, first, let's review some basic aspects about stress and the anatomy of sleep. ☾

[EXERCISE 1.1]

Self-Assessment: Poor Sleep Habits Questionnaire

Please take a moment to answer these questions based on your typical behavior. If you feel your sleep quality is compromised, consider that one or more of these factors may contribute to patterns of insomnia by affecting your physiology, circadian rhythms, or emotional thought processing. Although there is no key to determine your degree of insomnia, each question is based on specific factors associated with either a good night's sleep or the lack of it. Use each question to help you fine-tune your "sleep hygiene."

QUESTION	YES	NO
1. Do you go to bed at about the same time every night?		
2. Does it take you more than 30 minutes to fall asleep once in bed?		
3. Do you wake up at about the same time every day?		
4. Do you drink coffee, tea, or caffeinated soda after 6:00pm?		
5. Do you watch television from your bed?		
6. Do you perform cardiovascular exercise 3-5 times per week?		
7. Do you use your bed as your office (e.g., homework, balance checkbook, write letters, etc.)?		
8. Do you take a hot shower or bath before you go to sleep?		
9. Do you have one or more drinks of alcohol before bedtime?		
10. Are you engaged in intense mental activity before bed (e.g., exams, projects, reports, finances, taxes)?		
11. Is your bedroom typically warm or even hot before you go to bed?		
12. Does your sleep partner snore, become restless, etc. in the night?		
13. Is the size and comfort level of your bed satisfactory?		
14. Do you suffer from chronic pain while lying down?		
15. Is your sleep environment compromised by noise, light or pets?		
16. Do you frequently take naps during the course of a day?		
17. Do you take medications (e.g., decongestants, steroids, anti-hypertensives, asthma, anti-depressants)?		
18. Do you tend to suffer from depression?		
19. Do you eat a large, heavy meal right before you go to bed?		
20. Do you use a cell phone regularly, particularly in the evening?		

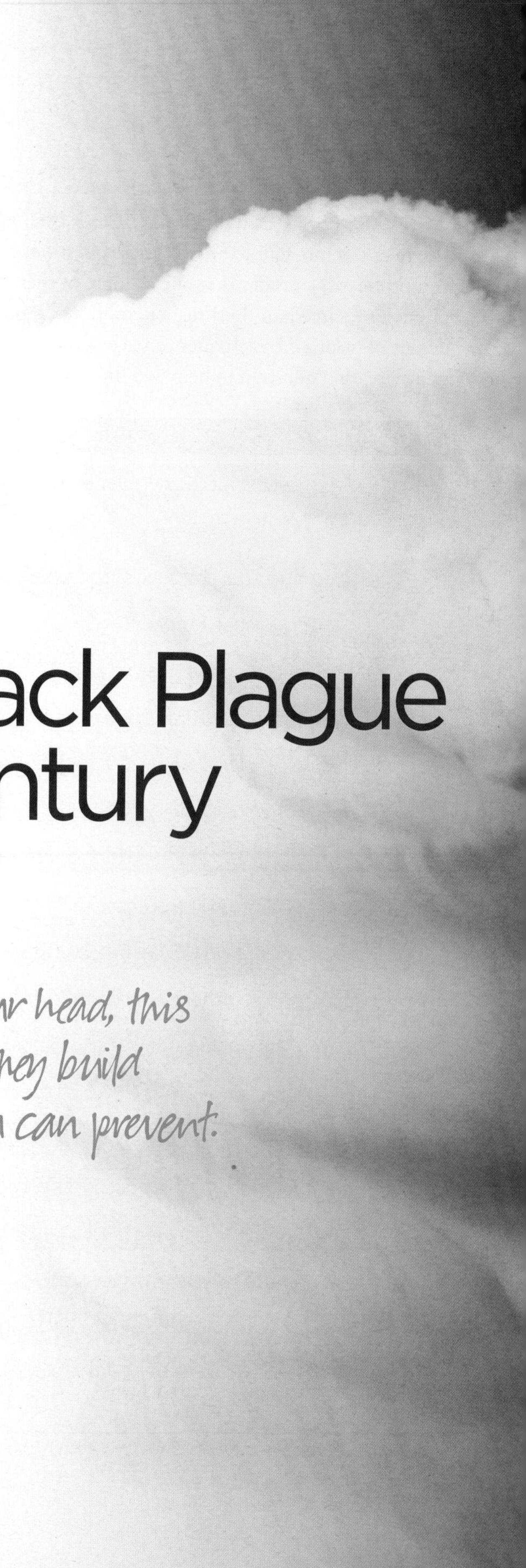

CHAPTER TWO

Stress: The Black Plague of the 21ST Century

That the birds fly above your head, this you cannot stop. But that they build nests in your hair, this you can prevent.

ANCIENT CHINESE PROVERB

"Storm Cloud" photograph by Brian Luke Seaward

CHAPTER TWO

Stress: The Black Plague of the 21ST Century

STRESS: THE BLACK PLAGUE OF THE 21ST CENTURY

Do you know the look on your face when someone tells you that you look tired? Tired eyes, perhaps the bags under the eyes, lack of vitality of the skin, even wrinkles—are all telltale signs of stress. That is the look that Kathy has lately. Over a latte grande she confides that no amount of make-up can cover up the stress she feels.

"My life is ridiculous. My mother has Alzheimer's, we need to put her in assisted living, but there are no vacancies yet, my daughter is applying to college and I am reviewing her applications, work is beyond demanding, my body aches because of Lyme disease, I cannot sleep, and I feel like I have no time for myself," she explains.

America leads the world in a number of ways, and not all of them are good, including our rapid, stressed-paced lifestyles. In the early 1990's, the World Health Organization (WHO) noticed a subtle, yet alarming trend around the planet. In one way or another, stress was taking a toll on people's physical health in nearly every country. In one of their annual reports they referred to stress as a "global epidemic." In the decades since this proclamation was made, researchers in the field of psychoneuroimmunlogy (mind-body medicine) have cited several definitive links between chronic stress and chronic disease, most notably (but not solely) the lingering effects of cortisol that suppress the immune system. Simply stated: When stress is not intercepted, the body becomes the battlefield for the war games of the mind. From the common cold to cancer, (not to mention a multitude of auto-immune diseases and a great many health related issues in-between), the stress and disease connection is not only quite real, it can be very deadly. In fact, take a closer look at the word disease (dis-ease) and you will see an obvious connection.

America leads the world in a number of ways, and not all of them are good, including our rapid, stressed-paced lifestyles.

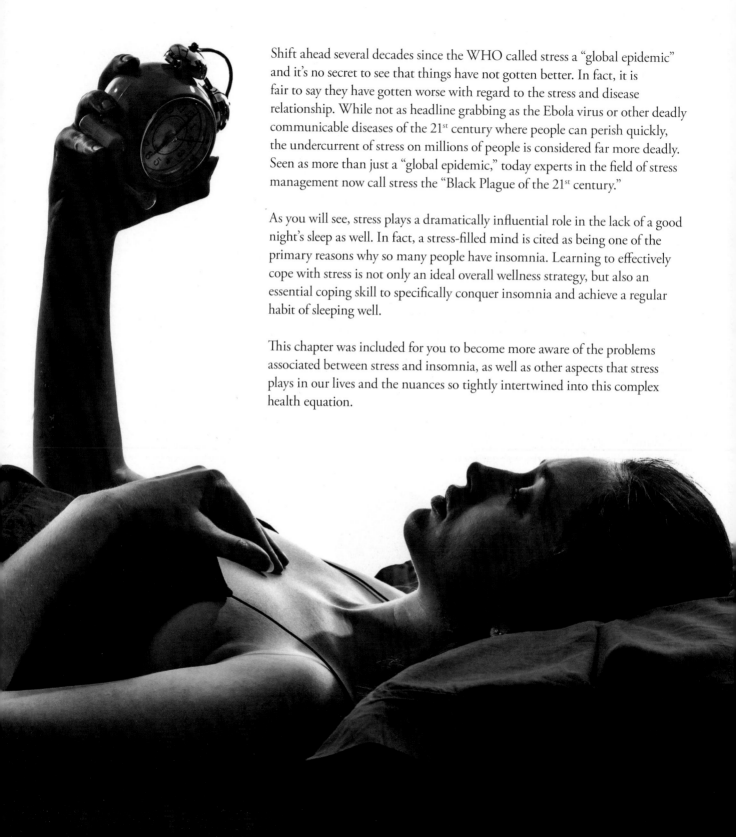

Shift ahead several decades since the WHO called stress a "global epidemic" and it's no secret to see that things have not gotten better. In fact, it is fair to say they have gotten worse with regard to the stress and disease relationship. While not as headline grabbing as the Ebola virus or other deadly communicable diseases of the 21st century where people can perish quickly, the undercurrent of stress on millions of people is considered far more deadly. Seen as more than just a "global epidemic," today experts in the field of stress management now call stress the "Black Plague of the 21st century."

As you will see, stress plays a dramatically influential role in the lack of a good night's sleep as well. In fact, a stress-filled mind is cited as being one of the primary reasons why so many people have insomnia. Learning to effectively cope with stress is not only an ideal overall wellness strategy, but also an essential coping skill to specifically conquer insomnia and achieve a regular habit of sleeping well.

This chapter was included for you to become more aware of the problems associated between stress and insomnia, as well as other aspects that stress plays in our lives and the nuances so tightly intertwined into this complex health equation.

This is Your Brain On Stress!

Every waking moment we take in thousands of bits of information through one or more of our five senses. Initially, each piece of information is routed through the lower brain as a means to judge if we are in physical danger. If there is no threat, we then process the information in a multitude of additional ways: curiosity, humor, puzzlement, analysis, etc. If a threat is determined, the body prepares for survival in what is commonly known as "fight or flight," also referred to as the "stress response." If you have ever been pulled over by the police for a speeding ticket, you no doubt have experienced first hand the fight or flight response; accelerated heart rate, increased blood pressure, increased breathing, tense muscles and an increased sweating response. This is your body's response to what it perceives as danger (in this case, an expensive speeding ticket). Truthfully speaking, your life is not in danger, but your body acts like it is.

A speeding ticket, however, is not the end of the world. Today we have very few physical threats such as saber-tooth tigers or burning buildings that must be evacuated, yet our bodies respond to all threats (mental, emotional, spiritual) as if every one is a physical danger (just in case we do need to move and move quickly). Some experts suggest that today the stress response is very antiquated for the safe and comfortable world in which we inhabit. Moreover, by having the stress response repeatedly "kick in" when danger is not imminent, we set the stage for some serious health-related problems. It's no secret that chronic stress and chronic disease go hand in hand. Left unresolved, stress kills.

Flight, Fright, Freeze!

Scientists have noticed that over the past two decades some people, under the threat of stress, neither fight nor flee. Like deer caught in the headlights of a rapidly approaching car, they just freeze. The "freeze response" is actually part of the flight response where, for some unknown reason, the neural message to move (flee) is corrupted and the flight response stalls out. We become frozen in time. Stress researchers have another name for the freeze response; "mental paralysis." In a world filled with sensory bombardment, in which an individual feels completely overwhelmed, mental paralysis is a common problem, and not just in the daylight hours. Mental paralysis resurfaces as one prepares for bed. The body is exhausted, yet like a rotating wheel in a hamster cage, the mind just keeps spinning, yet never going anywhere. An active mind, under the influence of stress, negates the opportunity for a good night's sleep.

> The "freeze response" is actually part of the flight response where, for some unknown reason, the neural message to move (flee) is corrupted and the flight response stalls out. We become frozen in time.

A Few Definitions of Stress

The topic of stress is colossal. Like an octopus, its tentacles spread over a number of aspects of our lives, so much so that several academic disciplines (e.g., psychology, physiology, sociology, anthropology, and theology, to name a few) have tried to understand it from their perspectives. As such, there are many different definitions for stress. Here are a few: From the field of physiology, stress is often defined as "wear and tear" on the body. All you need to do is think of a tension headache and realize that definition works well. From the field of psychology, we see that stress can be defined as the loss of emotional control (think road rage), or even the inability to cope with problems. From a spiritual perspective, stress is often defined as "the absence of inner peace." Quite true, indeed!

If you were to get all the stress experts in a room together and tell them no one can leave until they come up with a consensus of what stress is, you might hear them say this: "Stress is a 'perceived' threat (real or imagined) to one's mind, body, spirit or emotions." The term "perceived" is essential here because you can have two people in an identical situation, each with a different perception; one pleasant, one stressful. How we interpret the situation is key to dealing with it, and interpretations can certainly vary. Furthermore, as we all know, people can make mountains out of molehills, as expressed in this popular quote by Mark Twain, " I am an old man now, and I have known a great many problems in my life… most of which never happened."

Good Stress and Bad Stress

All stress is not created equal. Some stress is actually quite good for you. Gravity, an energetic force that helps keep bones strong is one example. So is inspiration; that unique personal energy to accomplish a goal or dream. Experts in the field of stress management speak of both good stress (also known as "eustress") and bad stress (also known as "distress"), but more commonly known simply as STRESS! Good stress is euphoric and exhilarating. It's where you want to reach your hands up in the sky and yell at the top of your lungs, "It doesn't get any better than this!" There is definitely an element of happiness and bliss with eustress. Even though you may also see an elevation in heart rate and blood pressure, the flood of "happy" hormones (e.g., serotonin and dopamine) and neuropeptides (e.g., beta-endorphins) associated with good stress typically negates the effects of the fight or flight response and soon everything returns to normal. In this case, normal means achieving a state of mental homeostasis.

With the use of brain scans, brain imaging and MRI's, medical science has looked deeply into the brain to understand its secrets; several of which have been revealed regarding the science of sleep.

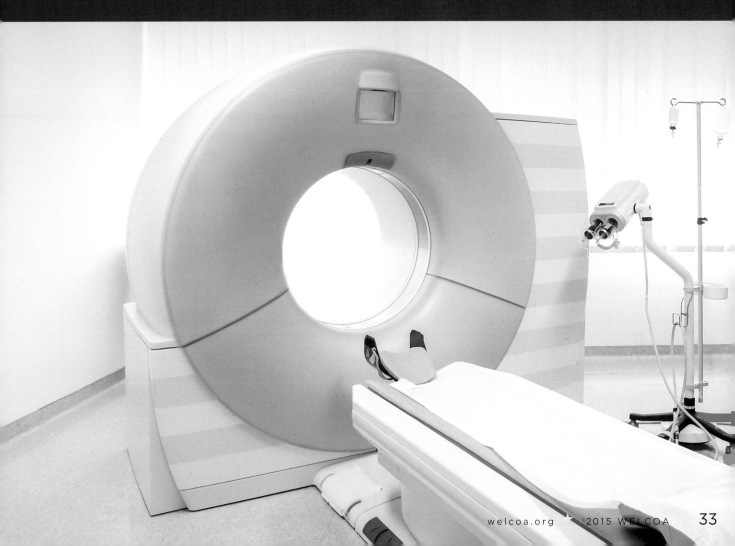

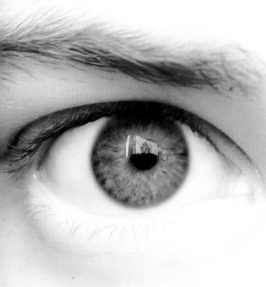

Anger is the fight response. Fear is the flight response.

Acute Stress and Chronic Stress

Experts who have studied the psychology and physiology of stress have delineated distress into two categories: Acute stress; that which is very intense, but rather short lived (about 20 minutes max), and chronic stress; that which is dramatically less intense, but can last for prolonged periods of time (e.g., days, weeks, months, even years). It is not usually acute stress that keeps one up at night, though this has been known to happen. By and large, stress-related insomnia is most often associated with chronic stress. Moreover, the duration of the stress might indicate the type of insomnia associated with it (i.e., intermittent or chronic insomnia, all of which will be discussed in more detail in Chapter 4).

The Stress Emotions: Anger and Fear

On the surface, it may seem like there are hundreds of emotions associated with stress, from panic to rage, but stated simply, there are two emotions associated with stress; anger and fear. All other stress-related emotions (e.g., guilt, anxiety, worry, impatience, frustration and envy, to name a few) are all aspects of anger or fear. In simple terms, anger is the fight response. Fear is the flight response. Calling to mind how complex stress can be, under stress, an individual can experience many emotions at one time, or in rapid succession. Because each of these stress emotions (anger or fear) is associated with physical survival, neither is considered bad when used for its intended purpose. On the contrary, anger and fear are considered healthy (in tiny amounts) to get you to safety. Problems arise when these emotions, fueled by the ego, last far longer than is necessary to get out of harm's way. One technique in stress management is to try to identify what emotion(s) you are feeling to the corresponding issue. Often times the cause of stress is an exaggeration, yet the emotions closely associated with it are very real. By taking time to reflect (process) the situation from different perspectives we can begin to minimize the emotional response and then work on a creative solution and resolution.

The Causes of Stress

Financial difficulties. Chronic health problems. Marriage troubles. Dead-end career path. The boss from hell. Perpetual lack of personal time. A rebellious teenager. A parent with Alzheimer's. The list of personal stressors that can keep us awake at night is nearly endless. Ask any person today what causes him or her stress and you will find the answers are quite varied, yet equally troublesome. Many of these personal problems have no quick solutions, yet ultimately they do have solutions.

From the definition of stress as a "perceived threat," it is easy to see that the ultimate cause of stress is not external matters as much as it is our perceptions and interpretation of the situation. Experts in the field of psychology will point out that the ego can easily make mountains out of molehills, and sabotage our best efforts for a good night's sleep. While making a list of stressors (e.g., problems, issues, concerns, dilemmas, etc.) is a good start in identifying what is on our mind, and what needs resolution, this is only half the solution in coping with stress. With regard to resolving issues, taming the ego is essential, as is using any and all effective coping skills to help achieve and maintain equilibrium of mind, body and spirit.

Effective Coping Techniques

Coping techniques fall into two categories: effective and non-effective. Many people are quite adept at the ineffective coping skills, perhaps because they all fall under the category of avoidance; drinking, drugs, self-medication, gambling, shopping, sex, even acts of violence. Quite honestly, these ineffective strategies only perpetuate stress. Conversely, effective coping strategies work to accomplish two goals: First, they shed light on the problem (often from different perspectives) to gain better insights on how to deal with it. Secondly, they lead you in the direction of resolution; finding some sense of peace with the situation. There are hundreds, if not thousands, of effective coping skills. Here are a few that have withstood the test of time, particularly with regard to getting a good night's sleep.

☾ **Journaling:** Sometimes sitting with a pen and pad of paper (or notebook) and writing down your thoughts and feelings before you go to bed is an ideal stress management strategy. Not only does journaling help you get these issues out of your head and down on paper, but it also helps give you some perspective on the situation. Consider placing a pen and pad of paper on your night stand. Before you turn out the lights, jot down (lists work just fine) whatever is on your mind, knowing that once on paper, you can revisit this list in the morning, once you have slept on it.

☾ **Time Management:** One reason why people claim not to get a good night's sleep is an over-packed schedule. The end result is that they often shave time off of the evening and

Humor is a proven way to lighten the load of a heavy mind. By looking for the humorous side to a situation (or even a non-related situation) it helps take the edge off of stress.

early morning hours of sleep to get caught up on a backlog of personal responsibilities. The consequences include cheating themselves of both quality and quantity of sleep. The irony is that by shaving off time from one's required sleep quota, the quality of work diminishes greatly. The essentials of good time management skills go well beyond inserting various obligations into your day planner. Time management often includes learning how to subtract things in your life that only add clutter. Time management also requires that you budget in essential personal time to relax and do nothing. No app will ever add more hours to the day.

☽ **Creative Problem Solving:** Many people, who claim not to sleep well, will tell you that they feel stuck or immobilized. A person without options sows the seeds for a stressful mind. Creative problem solving skills help you find options to any problem. As you become empowered with creative viable options (solutions) you move from victim to victor. Exercise 2.3 addresses the steps to the creative problem-solving process.

☽ **Reframing:** How do you turn lemons into lemonade? First to gain some perspective, you start by looking for the good side of a bad or difficult situation. Reframing invites you to put the problem in a different context, one that is non-threatening. It is empowering to realize you have the ability to choose your own thoughts. There is a wonderful adage used in stress management classes: "Every situation has a good side and a bad side: each moment you decide."

☽ **Humor:** You may wonder how laughing at your troubles can help solve them, but it's true. Humor is a proven way to lighten the load of a heavy mind. By looking for the humorous side of a situation (or even a non-related situation) it helps take the edge off of stress. Self-deprecating humor (making light of yourself, without sacrificing your self-esteem) is often recommended as well. Finally, building a tickler notebook (a compilation of funny jokes, pictures, birthday cards, etc.) is a great way to shift your mind away from the whirlpool of negativity that can keep you awake at night. Exercise 2.4 invites you to add some more humor in your life and not take yourself too seriously.

☾ **Acceptance:** Not all stressors can be reframed, laughed at, or creatively solved. As hard as it may be, some stressors simply have to be accepted as is. The serenity prayer is one of the best stress management programs (philosophy) summed up in 27 words: "God, grant me the serenity to accept the things I cannot change, the wisdom to change the things I can, and the wisdom to know the difference."

The Physical Symptoms of Stress

Stress may begin in the mind, but it rapidly moves through the central nervous system, starting in the brain (hypothalamus and amygdala). With the lightning speed of an electrical current, it spreads through the sympathetic nervous system to the muscles (in preparation for fight or flight). At the same time there is a flood of stress hormones activated to prepare the body for a wild display of metabolic activity (also in preparation for fight or flight). With the speed and dexterity of the sympathetic nervous system that innervates nearly all of the body's muscle tissue, it comes as no surprise that the most common symptom of stress is muscle tension, from headaches to lower back pain and much in between. The mind-body dynamic is as complex as it is amazing. When repetitive hormonal activity excites the corresponding target organ tissue (e.g., skin, stomach, lungs, heart, pancreas, liver, etc.), the specific organ with increased metabolic activity can become overworked and ultimately exhausted. An organ that becomes exhausted is a prime candidate for disease or illness (depending on the organ, possible death). As the expression goes, "the issues are in the tissues."

Excess sympathetic nervous activity can also interact with the immune system (to either suppress it or in some cases, accelerate it into overdrive, setting the stage for an auto-immune response). Many auto-immune diseases are described in the medical literature as "The body attacking the body." Lupus, Crohn's disease, rheumatoid arthritis, multiple sclerosis, and fibromyalsia are just a few classified as auto-immune diseases.

Physical exercise IS the fight or flight response fully realized. Just as the human body needs relaxation, it also needs physical exertion to keep the heart and lungs in prime shape, and the muscles well toned.

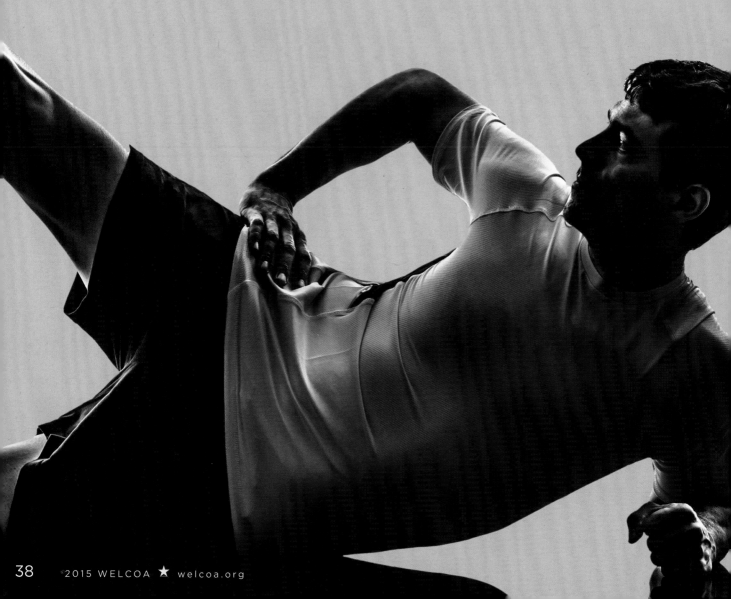

Effective Relaxation Techniques

Picture this: You are sitting in a hot jacuzzi, surrounded by soft-lit candles as your muscles melt under the foam of lavender sea salts. Or consider this: A massage therapist dims the lights, starts some relaxing music and begins to unravel the string of knots in your shoulders and upper back. Just like effective coping strategies for stress, there are many, many effective relaxation techniques. By some accounts, all effective coping techniques fall into one (perhaps several) of five categories: Sight, sound, taste, touch and smell. We take up thousands upon thousands of bits of information through one or more of our five senses and at times this can be overwhelming. Conversely, we can take in relaxing stimulation and return the mind and body to homeostasis. Here are a few of the most common time-honored relaxation techniques that promote inner tranquility:

☾ **Physical Exercise:** Let there be no doubt; physical exercise is stress. Physical exercise IS the fight or flight response fully realized. Just as the human body needs relaxation, it also needs physical exertion to keep the heart and lungs in prime shape, and the muscles well toned. We also know that when people complete a cardiovascular exercise session their heart rate and blood pressure lower and their body returns to homeostasis much quicker. People often associate regular physical exercise with weight loss or weight control, but one of the best benefits of physical exercise is a good night's sleep.

☾ **Hatha Yoga:** Hatha yoga is a daily practice of several repeated physical positions (called asanas) to help align the spine for better posture. By holding and repeating these postures (and stretching tight muscles that contribute to poor posture) this type of exercise has become a favorite for many people across the country. Hatha yoga, however, is more than mere muscle stretching. It is a metaphor to live your life in balance. Like physical rhythmic exercise, one of the benefits of Hatha yoga is a better night's sleep, according to various articles in the *Yoga Journal*.

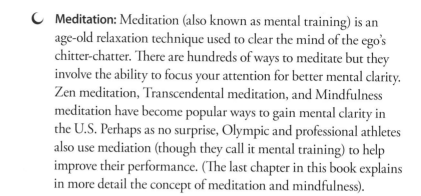

☾ **Meditation:** Meditation (also known as mental training) is an age-old relaxation technique used to clear the mind of the ego's chitter-chatter. There are hundreds of ways to meditate but they involve the ability to focus your attention for better mental clarity. Zen meditation, Transcendental meditation, and Mindfulness meditation have become popular ways to gain mental clarity in the U.S. Perhaps as no surprise, Olympic and professional athletes also use mediation (though they call it mental training) to help improve their performance. (The last chapter in this book explains in more detail the concept of meditation and mindfulness).

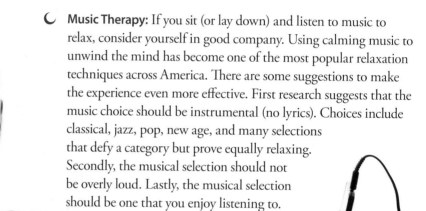

☾ **Music Therapy:** If you sit (or lay down) and listen to music to relax, consider yourself in good company. Using calming music to unwind the mind has become one of the most popular relaxation techniques across America. There are some suggestions to make the experience even more effective. First research suggests that the music choice should be instrumental (no lyrics). Choices include classical, jazz, pop, new age, and many selections that defy a category but prove equally relaxing. Secondly, the musical selection should not be overly loud. Lastly, the musical selection should be one that you enjoy listening to.

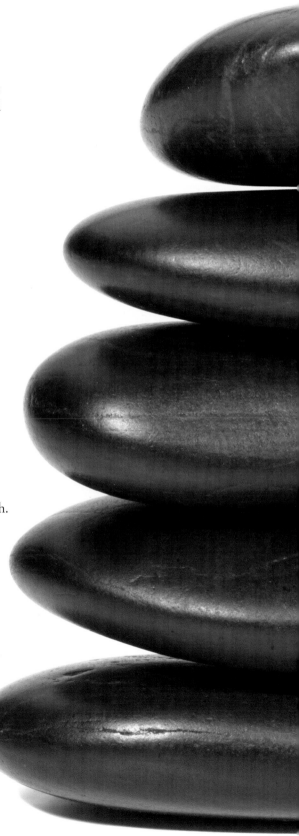

☾ **Tai Chi:** When most people think of meditation, they think of sitting still. Tai Chi is affectionately called "the moving meditation." Based on the dynamics of the softest of the Chinese martial arts, Tai Chi is best described as a progression of physical movements in which to align the body's core energy for optimal health. Not only does it improve posture and attention span, it also serves to align mind and body in normal daily activities and helps promote a good night's sleep.

☾ **Nutrition:** There are many foods that promote relaxation. When it comes to promoting a good night's sleep, there are also foods to avoid as day turns to night. One such food category is anything that contains caffeine (coffee, tea, sodas and chocolate). What are some foods to consume to promote a deeper sense of relaxation? Sleep experts often recommend sipping a cup of hot herbal tea before bed: herbs of choice include chamomile and lavender.

Balance: All Stress Begs for Resolution

Life without stress would be boring. Life with too much stress is exhausting (and potentially deadly). Somewhere between these two points is desirable balance. Perhaps as no surprise, this delicate but essential balance point is different for each person (based on personality, age, gender, and many, many other factors). The bottom line is this: All stress begs for resolution. This means that left unresolved, a problem will sabotage quality sleep and ultimately wreck havoc on your physical health. In the western culture, it is common to address the symptoms of a problem and ignore the root cause. This approach is commonly seen in the medical profession where a prescription is written or sought, yet the cause of the problem goes unaddressed. The best approach is a holistic one, where both causes and symptoms are addressed and effective coping skills and effective relaxation skills are employed to achieve and maintain a sense of balance. In a world where rapid-paced lifestyles will only increase the potential for stress, it behooves all of us to step back and take command of our lives. ☾

Life without stress would be boring. Life with too much stress is exhausting (and potentially deadly). Somewhere between these two points is desirable balance.

[EXERCISE 2.1]

Are You Stressed?

Although there is no definitive survey composed of 20+ questions to determine your level of stress, questionnaires do help increase awareness that, indeed, there may be a problem in one or more areas of your life (that things are out of balance). The following is a simple stress inventory to help you determine the level of stress/imbalance in your life. Read each statement and then mark either the word Agree or Disagree. Then count the number of "agree" points (one per question) and use the Stress Level Key to determine your personal stress level.

STATEMENT	AGREE	DISAGREE
1. I have a hard time falling asleep at night.	☐	☐
2. I tend to suffer from tension and/or migraine headaches.	☐	☐
3. I find myself thinking about finances and making ends meet.	☐	☐
4. I wish I could find more to laugh and smile about each day.	☐	☐
5. More often than not, I skip breakfast or lunch to get things done.	☐	☐
6. If I could change my job situation, I would.	☐	☐
7. I wish I had more personal time for leisure pursuits.	☐	☐
8. I have lost a good friend or family member recently.	☐	☐
9. I am unhappy in my relationship or am recently divorced.	☐	☐
10. I haven't had a quality vacation in a long time.	☐	☐
11. I wish that my life had a clear meaning and purpose.	☐	☐
12. I tend to eat more than three meals a week outside the home.	☐	☐
13. I tend to suffer from chronic pain.	☐	☐
14. I don't have a strong group of friends to whom I can turn.	☐	☐
15. I don't exercise regularly (more than three times per week).	☐	☐
16. I am on prescribed medication for depression.	☐	☐
17. My sex life is not very satisfying.	☐	☐
18. My family relationships are less than desirable.	☐	☐
19. Overall, my self-esteem can be rather low.	☐	☐
20. I spend no time each day dedicated to meditation or centering.	☐	☐

STRESS LEVEL KEY

Less than 5 points	You have a low level of stress and maintain good coping skills.
More than 5 points	You have a moderate level of personal stress.
More than 10 points	You have a high level of personal stress.
More than 15 points	You have an exceptionally high level of stress.

[EXERCISE 2.2]

Practicing the Art of Subtraction

Does your life feel cluttered with too much stuff? Are your garage and basement filled with "stuff" that you haven't used (or seen) in years? Are there people in your life who are so emotionally needy that when you see them, you want to run and hide? Are there things in your life that at first seemed to simplify your life and now they seem to be complicating it? If so, you might want to consider engaging in the Art of Subtraction (also known as "editing your life"), a time management technique to can help you remove clutter in your life.

I **Clutter!** Walk through your house or apartment and make a list of five things that fall in the category of personal clutter (this can include equipment, clothes, books, or anything lying on the floor). Once you have made this list, collect the things and consider giving them away to Goodwill or some other charitable organization.

1.

2.

3.

4.

5.

II **People!** Are there people in your life who take up time rather than contribute to your quality of life? Take inventory if you have any "friends" who seem to be a drain of your emotional energy. The next question to ask yourself is this: Do you drain other people's energy? Do you give as well as take in your relationships and friendships?

1.

2.

3.

III **Simplicity vs. Complexity!** We tend to bring things into our lives out of both interest and fear. What things are in your life right now that may have begun out of interest, but now you are ready to let go of? Another way to phrase this question is to ask yourself: What things in your life tend to add complexity rather than simplicity? Once you have identified three things, begin to ask yourself what you can do to subtract these things to bring your life back into balance.

1.

2.

3.

[EXERCISE 2.3]

Creative Problem Solving 101

There are several good ways to solve a problem! All you need to do is spend some time working at it from different directions until a number of viable solutions surface, and then choose the best one. The following is a time-tested strategic plan for creatively trying to solve problems and coming to a sense of resolution.

The Problem:

1 Define/Describe the Problem (please be as specific as you can):

    A.   How would a child see this problem?

    B.   How would an alien see this problem?

    C.   How would a 23rd century citizen see this problem?

    D.   How would you describe this problem to a person from a different culture?

2 Generating Great Ideas (List at least four viable ideas and one crazy, preposterous idea (X) to bring out the play factor):

    A.

    B.

    C.

    D.

    X.

3 Idea Selection and Refinement (Pick the best idea from above and explain WHY you think this is the best idea.):

    1.

    2.

    3.

4 Idea Implementation (Explain how you will put this idea into action. Make a brief, four-point outline of your action plan):

    A.

    B.

    C.

    D.

4 Evaluation and Analysis of "Action Plan" (How well did it work? What improvements would you make?):

[EXERCISE 2.4]

Comic Relief: Making a Tickler Notebook

Consider this! The average child laughs or giggles about 300 times a day. The typical adult laughs about 15 times a day. Research reveals that the average hospital patient never laughs at all. This assignment invites you to make a tickler notebook (3-ring notebooks work best), comprised of favorite jokes, photographs, birthday cards, love letters, Dear Abby columns, poems or anything else that brings a smile to your face. Keep the tickler notebook on hand, so if you are having a bad day, you can pull it out to help you regain some emotional balance. And, if you ever find yourself in the hospital for whatever reason, be sure to bring it along so that you can at least get your quota of 15 laughs a day.

The following are two jokes to help you form a critical mass of funny things to include in your notebook.

The New Boss

A company, feeling it is time for a shakeup, hires a new CEO. This new boss is determined to rid the company of all slackers. On a tour of the facilities, the CEO notices a guy leaning on a wall. The room is full of workers and he wants to let them know he means business! The CEO walks up to the guy and asks, "And how much money do you make a week?" Undaunted, the young fellow looks at him and replies, "I make about $200 a week. Why?"

The CEO hands the guy $1,000 and screams, "Here's a month's pay with benefits, now GET OUT and don't come back!"

Surprisingly, the guy takes the cash with a smile, and says, "Yes sir! Thank you, sir!" and leaves.

Feeling pretty good about his first firing, the CEO looks around the room and asks, "Does anyone want to tell me what that slacker did around here?"

With a sheepish grin, one of the other workers mutters, "Pizza delivery guy from Domino's."

This is the Bell Curve of Life

At age 4, success is…	not peeing in your pants.
At age 12, success is…	having friends.
At age 16, success is…	having a driver's license.
At age 20, success is…	having sex.
At age 30, success is…	having money.
At age 50, success is…	having money.
At age 60, success is…	having sex.
At age 70, success is…	having a driver's license.
At age 75, success is…	having friends.
At age 80, success is…	not peeing in your pants!

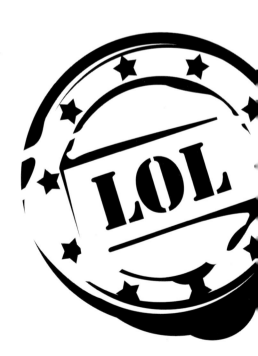

CHAPTER THREE

A Busy Mind: Digital Toxicity, FOMO and Digital Detox

Too much screen time damages the brain.

PSYCHOLOGY TODAY

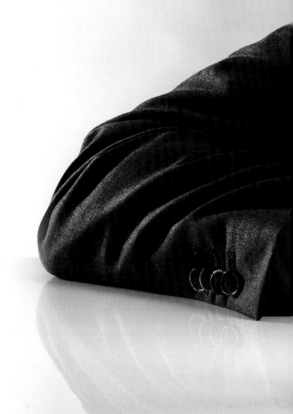

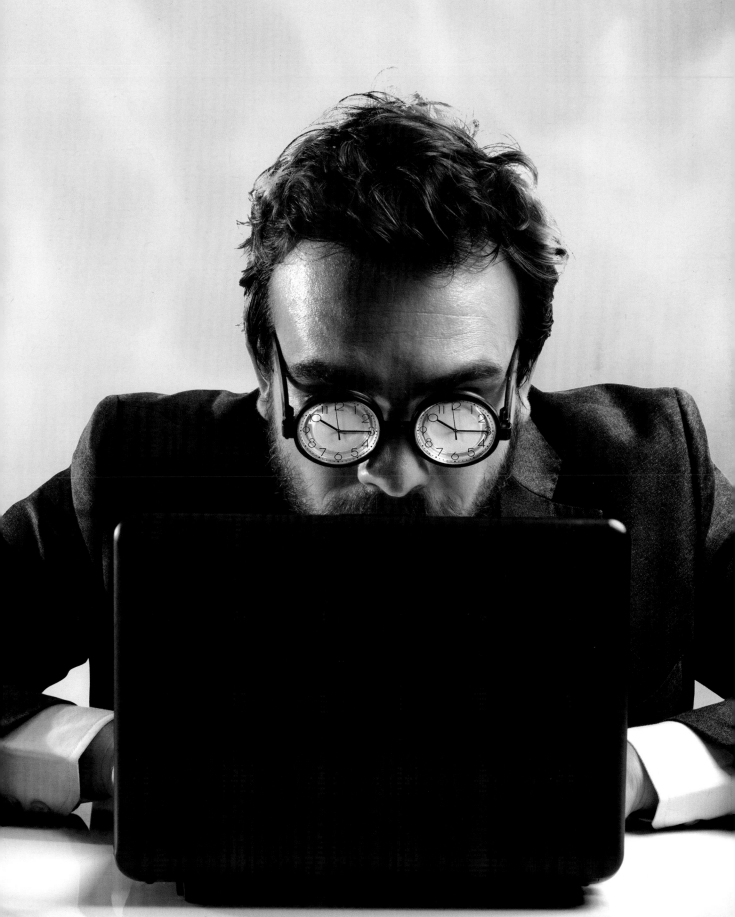

CHAPTER THREE

A Busy Mind: Digital Toxicity, FOMO and Digital Detox

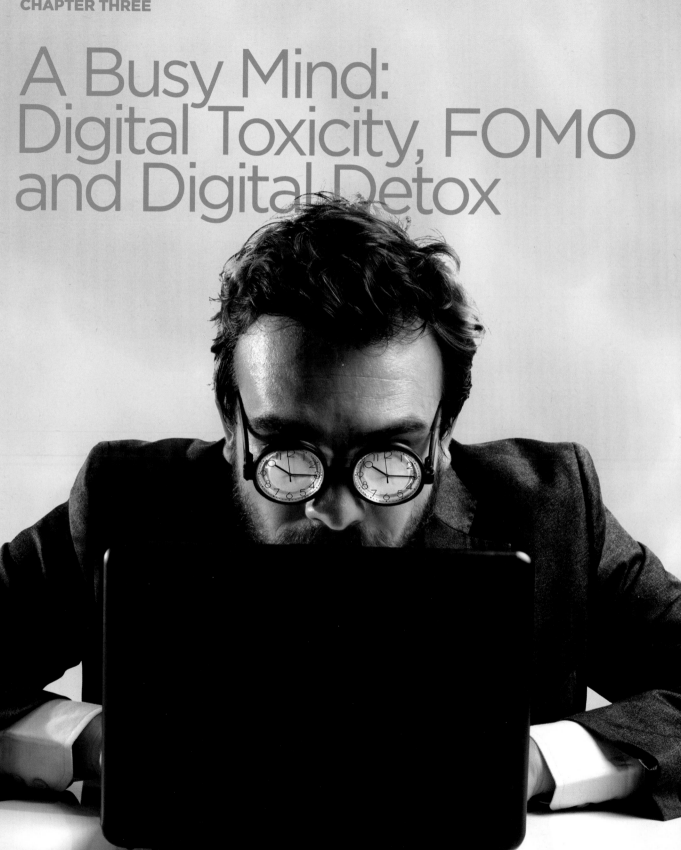

 welcoa.org

Brendan carries his cell phone with him everywhere, even to bed. "There's an alarm clock app," he says, with an innocent grin. Over dinner he excuses himself several times to answer incoming text messages. As a manager for an airline business, his hours go well beyond the typical 9 a.m. to 5 p.m. work schedule. "We move race horses, medical supplies, laboratory animals, all kinds of precious cargo. Heck, we've been known to ship the Queen's laundry across continents on occasion. The world of airfreight is a 24/7 business," he said. "I have to be honest with you. I swear to God, I haven't had a good night's sleep since I got this thing," he adds, holding the smart phone in his hand. Our conversation turned to the topic of digital toxicity. Brendan nods in agreement with everything.

Over a dinner conversation several weeks later, Brendan looks well-rested. "You were right about leaving my cell phone out of the bedroom. It has changed my life, my wife's too. I sleep like a baby all through the night now. I put the old alarm clock/clock radio back in to use. What a difference! Unplugging the WiFi each night has helped too, it's become a ritual: unplug from the world to gain some sanity. Who knew that a little piece of technology could wreak such havoc in the evening hours."

Welcome to a Culture of Distractions!

Do you flinch every time your cell phone or tablet "pings" with a text message, tweet, or email? Have you ever felt overwhelmed with a deluge of emails waiting for you at the start of each workday? Do you sit down to read a few Facebook posts or watch a YouTube video link for just a few minutes, and then realize that hours have disappeared in the blink of an eye? Does your spouse tell you that you spend more time with your smart phone than with him or her? Do you multi-task with your smart phone and tablet at all hours to stay connected to the world? If your response to any of these questions is an affirmative, congratulations, you are in good company with several common, perhaps questionable, high-tech habits, any of which will affect your quality of sleep.

It wasn't that long ago that our choices to communicate (e.g., U.S. mail or the AT&T home phone) as well as ways to retrieve news and entertainment were somewhat limited (e.g., three television networks, a handful of local radio stations and one phone number per household). Today, we have endless cable channels, unlimited varieties of entertainment options, and countless ways to communicate with each other, all of which has led to a daily tsunami of information overload. The experts have a name for this. They call it "digital toxicity." Perhaps as no surprise, the carry-over effect of digital toxicity in the daylight hours is that our minds become hard to turn off at night, when it's time to sleep. Technology is not bad. It is how we use it that can be problematic and questionable.

> Today, we have endless cable channels, unlimited varieties of entertainment options, and countless ways to communicate with each other, all of which has led to a daily tsunami of information overload.

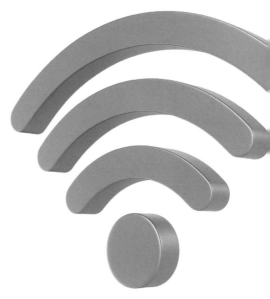

> ...we now live in a "culture of distractions;" countless people, friends, advertisers, networks and bites and bytes of information, all vying for our attention under a cacophony of digital noise.

It's no secret that the pace of life in the digital information age is fast and furious, and shows no signs of slowing down. Today, many people claim that they are overwhelmed as a result of a complicated alchemy of personal responsibilities, financial obligations and most notably, the never-ending demands of social media; texting, emails, Facebook updates, LinkedIn requests, Instagram and Snapchat posts or Twitter and Tumblr news feeds. Ads in current magazines often show a man (or woman) sitting with their feet up, glaring at their tablet or laptop screen with the headline: "Down time is the new uptime." The implied message is clear: Don't relax, don't unplug. Surf till you drop, then do it all over again. This short-term convenience to satisfy curiosity (and egos) has serious long-term implications on health, particularly one's sleep habits.

As has been noted by several experts who keep their finger on the metaphorical pulse of American society, we now live in a "culture of distractions;" countless people, friends, advertisers, networks and bites and bytes of information, all vying for our attention under a cacophony of digital noise. Over time, the end result is that our minds become well-groomed to perform with a minimal attention span-shifting focus like a ricochet ball in a racquetball court. In essence, our minds operate with an impaired ability to focus on anything longer than a few moments, yet at the same time the mind is constantly racing to see what else can feed it with new digital stimulation. Consequently, we have a perpetual fractured attention span (known as "monkey-mind"). Sociologists now suggest that the addiction to screen technology is the new social addiction of the 21st century. Once a big advocate of screen technology, MIT professor Sherry Turkle, author of the acclaimed book, *Alone Together,* now lectures about unhealthy behaviors associated with "digital toxicity."

How does digital toxicity affect sleep? According to the National Institute on Sleep in Arlington, Virginia, we now have an invasion of technology in the bedroom with smart phones, tablets and multiple screens negatively affecting both the quantity and quality of sleep. The implications for both work productivity and overall health are daunting.

FOMO: Fear of Missing Out

When Aldous Huxley wrote his classic novel, *Brave New World* in 1932, he envisioned an advanced, high-tech society where people were, in essence, socially numbed by the intoxicating effects of a wonder drug. However, just as cautions are forecasted in various sci-fi movies, serious and imminent dangers lurk beneath the utopian promise of a better life. What Huxley illustrated so clearly was the ego's pleasure sensation to a mind-altering stimulus. It could be argued quite favorably that indeed the Internet (and all the means to access it) is Huxley's mythical wonder drug of the 21st century. Left undisciplined, the ego becomes the gateway to addictive behavior. And the ego, it turns out, has an insatiable hunger for digital stimulation. Just as rapidly as these technologies and apps appear, so too, do names to describe behaviors associated with them. Experts in the field of sociology and psychology note the addictive quality to the Internet with the new term, "screen addictions." Fear of Missing Out (FOMO) is a new term to describe one rationale behind screen addictions; the ego's quest to be in the know at all times. Knowledge is power, and the ego loves power. Like other addictions, those associated with digital technology not only negatively impact the relationships within family dynamics and friends, they feed the ego's need for control in the new voyeuristic, 24/7, on-demand world of instant gratification. Paradoxically, in such situations, we give our power away. In essence, we become a slave to the technology master.

Inundated by a tsunami of text messages, Facebook posts, LinkedIn updates, multiple emails, Skype or FaceTime conversations, countless tweets, and a multitude of YouTube links, the average person is so distracted with bits and bytes of information that it's not only affecting work performance, it's affecting work relationships, marriages, leisure habits, sleep habits, driving habits and without a doubt, one's overall health status. Moreover, the exact toll of techno-stress may be hard to measure, but the social impact, from poor eye contact during face-to-face conversations to poor social etiquette, is unquestionable. The negative impact on health and wellness (mind, body, spirit and emotions) is undeniable. This impact becomes all the more catastrophic when people drive and text. The dangers are compounded when people do this during work and kill scores of people, as was observed in the catastrophic 2014 Madrid and NYC train collisions where it was discovered that the train conductors were texting.

> Experts in the field of sociology and psychology note the addictive quality to the Internet with the new term, "screen addictions."

Digital Dementia

Have you ever sat down in your car, entered an address into your GPS device, then driven off, letting the wonders of satellite technology navigate you toward your intended destination—only to find that the next time you set out to drive to the same destination, you had no idea how to get there? Spelling and grammar, once a staple of grade school English classes are now as easy to forget as the multiplication tables because of the sophisticated software that autocorrects spelling for us (although not without some humorous misgivings with text messaging). Another example has become a favorite Facebook/Twitter post that has gone viral many times over:

Daughter   Mom, where are you?

Mother   Honey, I just left Walmart. Be home soon. Why?

Daughter   Mom, you brought me to Walmart with you.

Mother   Uh-oh, sorry, I'll be right there.

Again, welcome to the brave new world of digital toxicity. As we rely more and more on savvy technology, we forfeit our ability to learn and memorize important facts, thus making us more reliant on it, making short- and long-term memory skills dull. The term used to describe this forfeiture of memory is called "Digital Dementia" and it has become more and more prevalent throughout the American society. Once again, technology is not bad; it is how we use it at times that becomes questionable.

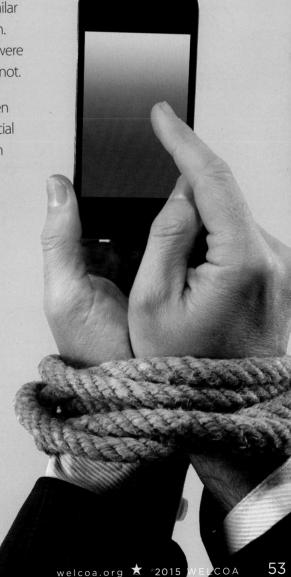

A BUSY MIND: A CLOSER LOOK AT "DIGITAL DEMENTIA"

With the world of information at our fingertips, can having access to so much information be a hindrance to memory rather than an asset? The answer appears to be a definitive YES! In an article titled, *A Smart Thing That Makes you Stupid,* investigative reporter, Ron Friedman, cites a series of studies that reveals the problem with being on-line with a smart phone all the time. In the first study, two groups of people were given a task; one group was allowed to have their cell phones within an arm's reach (on the table where they were working). The second group had no access to their smart phones. When the results were tabulated the group of people with access to their smart phones did 20% worse than the control group. In a similar study, people were asked to participate in a face-to-face conversation. Those who had a smart phone within reach found the person they were in conversation with boring, while those without a smart phone did not.

The results showed that when one's focus is split (distracted) between a task and the anticipation of a text message, email, phone call or social media post (the opposite of "undivided attention") memory function is compromised. For information to be transferred from short-term to long-term memory, the brain requires periods of rest. When people are glued to their devices, there is no time for the brain to rest and hence, shift necessary information from short-term to long-term memory.

Likewise, in a study to determine if the process of taking handwritten lecture notes was superior or inferior to memory formation, when compared to taking notes on a computer, results showed that old fashioned note taking is far superior. As people listened and wrote by hand, they were forced to synthesize the information rather than merely transcribe it digitally, hence they were better able to demonstrate memory recall.

Friedman has these suggestions to avoid digital dementia: 1) keep smart phones off desks, 2) banish email and text alerts, and 3) schedule distraction-free periods each day.

Facebook is now cited as the third leading cause for divorce.

Digital Obesity

Obesity has been a health concern in America for well over three decades, but this concern has become confounded with the advent of digital screen technology. Today, fewer and fewer people are exercising. Instead, people are consumed with sitting and surfing the Internet, something very hard to do while you are walking, jogging or swimming. The new phrase in corporate wellness programs goes like this: "Sitting is the new smoking of the 21st century." Health professionals who see the link between "serial sitting" and serial screen habits merely call it "Digital Obesity": The accumulation of excess weight due to the sedentary lifestyle promoted by fascination with screen technology. The human body was never designed to sit for 8-12 hours a day. Although there are many factors associated with obesity, we can add a new risk factor to the list: screen addictions.

Here are some "Brave New Digital World" facts to consider:

☾ Research now reveals that the average person checks his or her email 37 times per hour.

☾ A 2010 study by Microsoft revealed that the average person receives over 110 emails per day and it takes over 15 minutes to refocus from the distraction of a single email.

☾ People cite more than 50 emails per day as "email stress," with many people saying that reading and responding to email becomes a distraction to getting their job done.

☾ Facebook is now cited as the third leading cause for divorce.

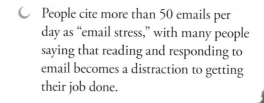

☾ Vacations were once a means to leave office work behind, but now people take their laptops, smart phones, and tablets with them everywhere, never allowing for downtime. Many national parks are fighting the urge to install WiFi in the campgrounds yet visitors are demanding it.

☾ A Manpower study revealed in 2010 that over 50% of employees never leave the office cubicle for lunch; the vast majority sits behind a keyboard never getting any exercise, natural sunlight or even fresh air.

☾ Each tweet, ping or "you've got mail" voice is associated with the release of dopamine (a chemical neurotransmitter) associated with euphoria; the feel-good hormone.

☾ The Kaiser Family Foundation found that 8-18 year olds spend over seven hours per day with entertainment media (video games, TV, apps, etc.).

☾ People who drive and text message show the same amount of distraction and poor reaction time as someone with a 0.08 blood alcohol level (the same demarcation as a drunk driver).

☾ The repeated use of technology makes people less patient and more forgetful.

☾ Sociologists cite screen addictions as a significant reason for the decline of civility in America.

☾ In 2011, the World Health Organization (WHO) issued a statement regarding the use of cell phones, electromagnetic fields and micro wave dangers associated with brain tumors, particularly with people under the age of 22 whose brains have not yet formed completely.

☾ The micro waves of cell phones and screen light is now known to interfere with brain physiology associated with sleep.

The Kaiser Family Foundation found that 8-18 year olds spend over seven hours per day with entertainment media (video games, TV, apps, etc.).

Research now reveals that the vibrations emitted from cell phones (and WiFi routers) greatly compromise the ability to produce Melatonin. When melatonin production is compromised, so is one's ability to sleep.

ELF's: Another Type of Digital Toxicity

In 1990, Robert Becker, MD, wrote a book, *Cross Currents,* warning Americans about the inherent dangers of electrical pollution, specifically ELF's (Extremely Low Frequency vibrations) generated from 60Hz electrical currents. Based on the laws of physics (entrainment and the conservation of energy) objects in close proximity tend to vibrate together. Noting the connection between high voltage power lines and the prevalence of cancer, Becker made the case, backed up by basic physics, that ELF vibrations (also known as micro waves) begin to destroy/mutate DNA, thus setting the stage for cancer. Cell phones have reignited this warning, primarily due to the close proximity of cell phones to one's head while in use. In 2010, Devra Davis wrote the acclaimed book, *Disconnect,* citing the research about cell phones and brain and throat cancer. Research now reveals that the vibrations emitted from cell phones (and WiFi routers) greatly compromise the ability to produce melatonin. When melatonin production is compromised, so is one's ability to sleep.

Smart phones have become essential in 21st century life. They are not going to go away any time soon, but we can be smart about how we use them. Ear pieces are highly recommend, but better yet, using the speaker phone feature on wireless and cordless phones is ideal so that the phone itself is not close to your head. Moreover, cell phones do not belong in the bedroom, and they should not be used as alarm clocks. Invest in a basic alarm clock.

The Need for Digital Detox

Let's state the obvious: Screen technology is exciting, amazing, yet without healthy boundaries, potentially dangerous. As the expression goes, everything in moderation. The mind (and the organ of choice it uses, the brain) were never meant to be over-stimulated with sensory bombardment every day, all day long. To repeat some vital information from Chapter 1, the mind not only craves, but needs homeostasis; repeated periods of rest and relaxation. Correspondingly, the brain needs time to detox. Both of these can occur simultaneously during quality sleep. Sleep is not a luxury. It is an essential component to health, wellness and longevity.

Digital detox begins with an awareness that time away from screen technology is not only good, it's crucial to your physical and mental health. It includes establishing healthy boundaries with the use of all screen technologies as well as dedicated time to meditate each day as a means to cleanse the mind of information overload.

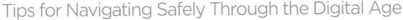

Tips for Navigating Safely Through the Digital Age

It's an understatement to say that stress and technology are an inseparable fact of life, particularly when things don't work the exact moment you need them, or when computers crash, smart phone batteries need recharging at crucial times or WiFi signals are weak. Regardless of the many reasons why stress and technology are forever linked, here are some time-tested tips for maintaining a sense of balance with the conveniences we have become so reliant upon in our brave new world.

1 PRACTICE HEALTHY BOUNDARIES

Setting healthy boundaries with technology is as important as honoring healthy boundaries with eating habits, finances and relationships. Given the pervasiveness of screen-based gadgets, perhaps even more so. There is no doubt that screen addictions are very real. Checking emails 37 times per hour, or constantly looking at Facebook is nothing short of an obsessive/compulsive act. Healthy boundaries with smart phones includes turning them off (completely) during staff meetings, meals at restaurants, meals at home, in movie theaters and of course, driving. Consider making it a habit not to check email until after 9:00 a.m. Make it a habit to only check Facebook at the end of each day, not 500 times in the course of each day.

Healthy boundaries are constructs of appropriate behavior you live by, based on your life values. Moreover, it's not enough to create healthy boundaries, you have to enforce them as well, otherwise feelings of victimization ensue. Create healthy boundaries and stick to them. Remember the motto: "Once a victim, twice a volunteer."

2 KEEP A "TECH-FREE" BEDROOM

Sociologists have noted a parallel increase of computer/smart phone use and insomnia (remember, over half of Americans claim to sleep poorly each night). The effect of a sleep-deprived workforce cannot be understated; work productivity (not to mention one's health) is greatly compromised. The National Institute of Sleep now calls this "The invasion of technology in the bedroom." Melatonin, the sleep hormone, is produced in the pineal gland as natural light diminishes and ambient temperature decreases. Without the proper amount of melatonin your quality of sleep is

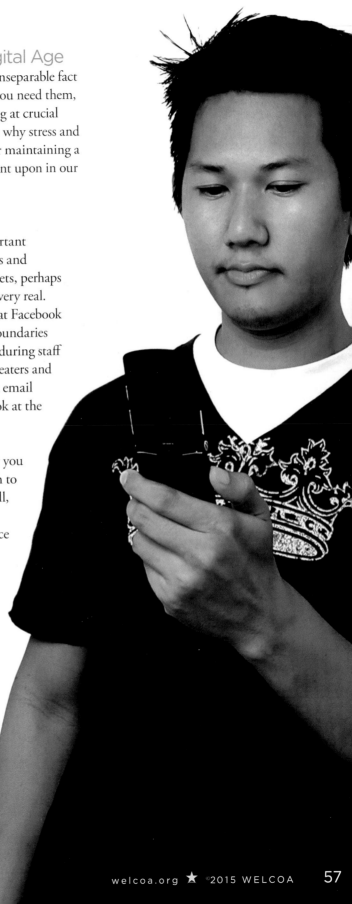

...despite all the wonders of technology, there will never be an app to make more hours in the day. Declare your bedroom a "technology-free zone" and honor this healthy boundary.

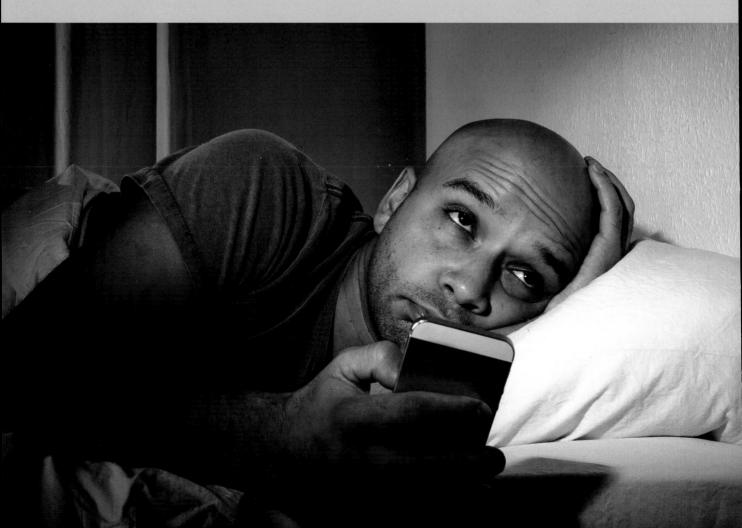

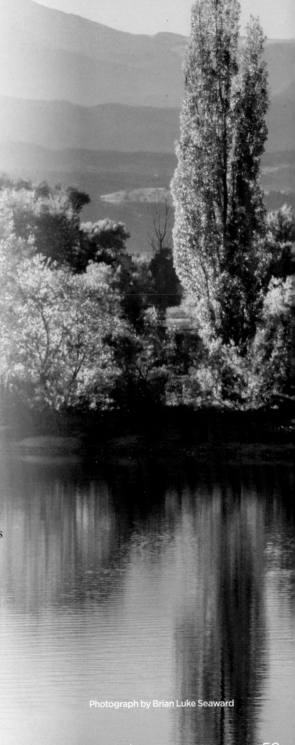

at risk. The pineal gland, which synthesizes melatonin, is light sensitive. Whereas overhead lights for reading will affect melatonin production, the light from backlit computer screens is directed onto the face and impacts melatonin to a much greater degree. The use of technology in the bedroom makes for bad sleep hygiene (see Chapter 5). Moreover, despite all the wonders of technology, there will never be an app to make more hours in the day. Declare your bedroom a "technology-free zone" and honor this healthy boundary. Remember, the bedroom has one function: Sleep (OK, possibly two functions, if you include sex).

3 MAINTAIN A MEDIA CURFEW

Just like curfews given to children with television watching or a designated time to return home from an evening school event, curfews are a great behavior to practice this moderation principle with screen technology. Considering the effects that smart phones and screen devices have on the production of melatonin, consider turning off all screen devices after a set time (e.g., 8:00 p.m.). This will allow your brain chemistry (melatonin/serotonin) to return to proper function several hours before embarking on a good night's sleep.

4 UNPLUG THE WIFI BEFORE YOU GO TO BED

According to research, the ELF (Extremely Low Frequency) micro waves from the WiFi router can negatively affect the production of melatonin. For this reason you may wish to consider unplugging or turning off the power to the WiFi each night before you go to bed. If you do have issues with falling asleep, try this for a week and see if you notice a difference.

5 SPEND QUALITY TIME DAILY OUTSIDE IN NATURE

Sunlight. Warm breezes. The smells of fresh cut grass. Flowering trees. Spring rain and the sound of song birds. Nature has many healing qualities, from the colors to the scents to the symphony of sounds of Mother Earth. Nature has a way to recalibrate our body's physiological clock through the sympathetic resonance of circadian rhythms. Make a habit of getting outside each day, every day to reconnect with nature.

6 BEST TO OPT FOR IN-PERSON COMMUNICATIONS

Communication experts are at a loss to explain all the ways to communicate these days. Teens prefer text messaging. Adults (over 35) prefer phone calls and emails. Adults over 55 prefer phone calls mostly.

Photograph by Brian Luke Seaward

> Sociologists have noticed a disturbing trend over the past decade, now called the "age of narcissism": people are extremely rude and social manners have become a rare commodity.

Experts now see that due to the dynamics of the digital age, social skills, particularly face-to-face communication skills, are sorely lacking. The end result is stress from miscommunication. Moreover, it is easy to avoid people through the use of smart phones and emails. It is not uncommon today for people to break up from an intimate relationship with a text message or quit a job with an email. Unlike face-to-face communication, the ability to misinterpret text messages and the like is not only easy, it's quite common. In 2011, the French company ATOS banned emails altogether. Others companies now require their employees not to email on Fridays in the hopes to foster more face-to-face contact. Smart idea. The lack of face-to-face contact fosters less empathy, and more mistrust, cynicism, and backstabbing; traits not conducive to a healthy work environment. Remember this axiom. The three keys to a successful business are: communication, communication and communication.

7 AVOID MULTITASKING ERRORS

While you may feel more productive doing several things at a time, the research shows that when your concentration is divided, quality suffers and the number of accidents/mistakes increases dramatically. Effective multitasking is a fallacy. In the case of texting while driving, people have been killed. Get in the habit of completing a task from start to finish without diversions such as constantly checking social media updates. If you catch yourself double dipping into other responsibilities, stop, take a deep breath and redirect your thoughts to one task and then finish it. Keep your mind focused on one thing at a time. Remember that distractions compromise quality work, no matter what you are doing. Successful multitasking is a myth!

8 HONOR THE RULES OF CIVILITY

Sociologists have noticed a disturbing trend over the past decade, now called the "age of narcissism": people are extremely rude and social manners have become a rare commodity. While the lack of manners may not be due to outright malice, the lack of civility is disturbing to many. Rude drivers, annoying dinner patrons, and inappropriate online behavior (web page rants, Facebook postings, emails and texting) have become the norm. The backlash of such behavior puts people on the social defense, raising the threshold of social stress.

Placing importance on yourself over your co-workers, colleagues, family or unsuspecting bystanders is an increasing phenomenon. The end result is an over-stressed population who feels slighted time after time to the point of general frustration. It's rude to answer a phone call during dinner. It's rude (and deadly) to text while driving. It's disrespectful to post inappropriate comments and photos on Facebook (much less have private arguments on a public forum). It's uncouth to talk on the cell phone while in the bathroom. Not long ago, manners were taught by parents (and teachers) to children. Yet the influx of social media and technology that has invaded our lives has also created poor modeling, mostly by parents to children, who in turn have grown up experiencing mild rudeness as socially acceptable behavior. While it's not your job to be the civility police, you can begin by modeling the highest form of politeness to everyone in your environments, starting with home and work.

9 CHOOSE QUALITY OVER CONVENIENCE

When polled about their behavior, people will often cite convenience as the reason why they talk on the cell phone while driving, or type on their keypads while talking on their cell phones. In the rush to get things done, instant gratification now rules! The irony is that quality often suffers at the expense of convenience. Ask any spouse who confides that their spouse spends more time talking on their cell phone than in a face-to-face conversation with them.

10 LEAVE THE OFFICE DURING THE LUNCH HOUR

It's no secret that Americans live a sedentary lifestyle; a lifestyle that has become even more so as technology has become so invasive in our lives. Let it be known that humans were never meant to sit down for six to eight straight hours per day and bang away on a keypad or have their eyes glued to a screen device all day (and night) long. Cardiovascular exercise is imperative each day. Make a habit to leave the technology behind and walk, jog, swim, bike, anything without the electronic leash of the Internet. Not only will your mind thank you for the break in sensory bombardment, but your body will thank you for flushing the stress hormones (e.g., cortisol) and setting the stage for a stronger immune system, a stronger cardiovascular system and a better night's sleep.

11 MAKE A DAILY HABIT OF MINDFUL MEDITATION

There is no magic pill for mental health, but a habit of meditation comes very close. As explained in the next chapter, engaging in a regular practice of meditation serves as a great way to help promote mental homeostasis. The benefits are quite conclusive. Meditation is a great way to create mental clarity. People have had

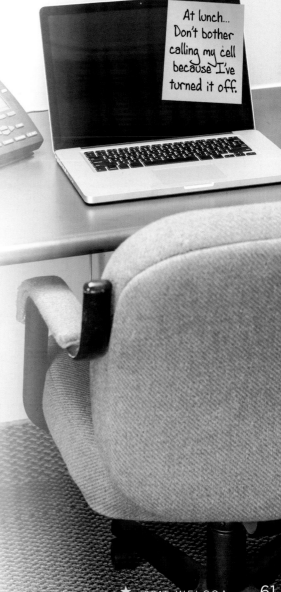

Make a habit to leave the technology behind and walk, jog, swim, bike, anything without the electronic leash of the Internet.

At lunch... Don't bother calling my cell because I've turned it off.

> The consensus is in: technology is great. It's just how we use it that makes us a master or a slave. A wise person knows the difference.

wandering minds long before the microprocessor was invented, millennia before smart phones and tablets. A wandering mind is closely associated with a powerful ego prowling the vicinity looking to distinguish various sensory stimulation as either friend or foe. Technology didn't create a wandering mind, but it sure does enhance the wandering, as anyone who has surfed the Internet or scrolled through countless Facebook postings for hours can attest. The practice of meditation has one purpose: to domesticate the ego, specifically the ego's countless distractions of negative thoughts. No matter what kind of meditation is practiced, the purpose is to increase one's concentration skills which then leads to an increased awareness. Athletes know the secret of meditation (they refer to it as "mental training") because they know that the slightest distraction during a competition can mean defeat; poor performance. In the business world, poor performance equates to poor work productivity. The "corporate athlete" needs meditation skills as much, if not more, than the professional athlete.

The skill of meditation teaches the practitioner to not only observe one's thoughts, but to observe oneself observing one's thoughts. This is called "mindfulness," and it is the tool to cultivate one's conscience. It also comes in handy when honoring the rules of civility. Meditation is as simple as closing your eyes and focusing on your breathing for several minutes. As distracting thoughts arise, simply let these go as you exhale. No matter how bored you may become, stick with this practice as a way to discipline your mind. Once you have domesticated the ego, you have mastered the power of the mind and the world is your oyster. As a side note, many people confide that they check emails, Facebook updates, voicemail and text messages because they are bored. Boredom is another form of distraction. Meditation: It's not what you think!

Slave or Master?

When technology combines with the dynamics of human psychology, a strange dilemma occurs. Technology always starts off as a means to improve our lives and serve us, with the inherent promise of adding hours of blissful leisure. This seldom happens. Instead, unknowingly, what first begins as a position of "master," quickly reverses to a subtle form of "slavery." We become hostage to the wonders of technology, ultimately giving our power away. Mastery requires a combination of will power and common sense; qualities we each have, but like muscles, need to be exercised regularly. The consensus is in: technology is great. It's just how we use it that makes us a master or a slave. A wise person knows the difference. ☾

[EXERCISE 3.1]

Slave or Master: The Internet Addiction Survey

A new social addiction has appeared on the scene, and it has ruined friendships, marriages, grade point averages, meetings and taught little children that smart phones and tablets are more important than they are. By some accounts, the Internet has magnified the human need of acceptance; the need to feel needed. Access to the Internet is now a public utility, and has become a part of everyday life, yet like a powerful black hole, one can become lost to the point of derailing one's life and those in one's immediate orbit including family, friends and co-workers. Are you a master or slave to the Internet?

RATE EACH STATEMENT: 1 = RARELY/NEVER 2 = OCCASIONALLY 3 = FREQUENTLY 4 = OFTEN 5 = NEARLY ALWAYS	
1. One of the first things I do each morning is check text messages, emails, Facebook updates or other websites of interest.	
2. Even though I might just check in briefly with social media sites, I end up online for longer than I plan, sometimes for hours.	
3. Although it might be considered illegal, I have been known to text while driving.	
4. I check Facebook or Google Plus comments and emails several times an hour each day.	
5. I become fidgety when I cannot pull out my smart phone or iPad to check messages, text messages, or social media updates.	
6. I commonly pull out my mobile device during a conversation with friends and check something on Google/social media sites.	
7. I post updates then repeatedly check to see who "likes" and comments on them, as well as frequently comment on other posts.	
8. I am easily distracted surfing the Internet, sometimes forgetting what I originally went online for.	
9. I can feel agitated/depressed when I cannot access my smart phone (e.g., dead battery, dead zone, etc.) for long periods of time.	
10. In the course of a typical day, I end up spending more time online than real time contact with friends, family and peers.	
11. I tend to get aggravated when I get interrupted while online.	
12. Online activities have a priority over work and many home responsibilities.	
13. Life without social networking, texting and web-surfing would be extremely boring, even unhappy.	
14. I quickly check email, Facebook or other social networking sites before meetings, appointments, etc.	
15. I have a hard time turning my cell phone/smart phone off.	
16. Friends and family comment about my online use.	
17. I become defensive when people comment on my use of the Internet.	
18. My sleep time has decreased since smart phones, tablets, etc. have come into my life.	
19. I watch TV, listen to the radio or do other things while online.	
20. The last thing I do before I got to sleep is check text messages and social media site updates.	
TOTAL	

Key: Score your answers by adding the points for each question for a grand total. The higher your score, the greater your level of addiction and the issues and concerns associated with Internet use or what is now commonly called, "screen addictions." Please use the following scale to help measure your score.

10-39 points   Normal online use. Keep in mind that normal is not always healthy.

40- 69 points   Internet activity leans in the direction of Internet addiction and healthy boundaries with Internet use are a good idea.

70-100 points   The amount of time you spend online is associated with addictive behaviors and thought should be given to changing this behavior with a practice of strong healthy boundaries.

CHAPTER FOUR

The Anatomy of Sleep

Sleep is the golden chain that ties health and our bodies together.

THOMAS DEKKER

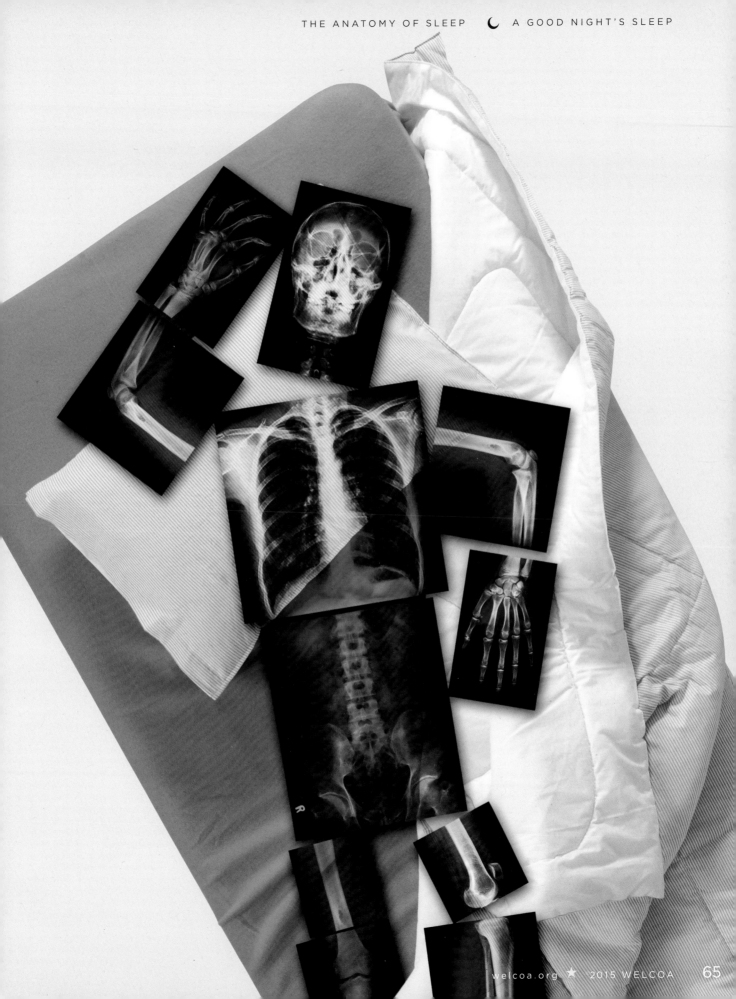

CHAPTER FOUR

The Anatomy of Sleep

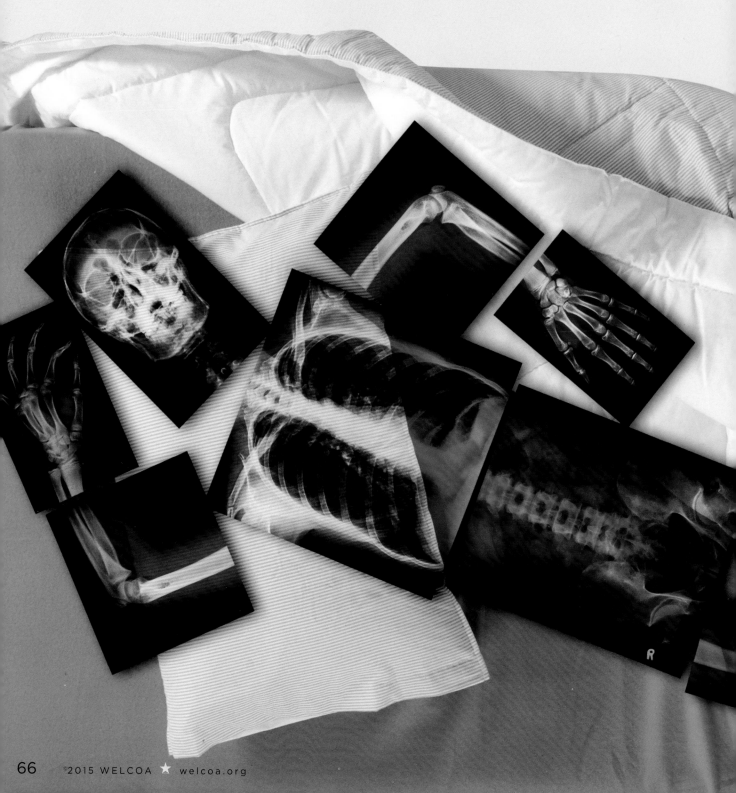

The sleep patterns of humanity are very different today than those of your great-grandparents who never knew the pleasures of electrical outlets, lamps, and power lines. Before the advent of electricity (and the utility bills that came with it), sleep behaviors were starkly different. Keep in mind that prior to 1900, most people lived an agrarian lifestyle; they read by candle light or oil lamps and heated their homes with wood or coal. Some people even brought farm animals inside to provide additional heat. Moreover, the typical home didn't have indoor plumbing (if you think waking up in the night to pee now is tough, consider that!) As such, most people didn't sleep undisturbed straight through the night. An interrupted night's sleep was a given. In his book, *At Day's Close, Night in Times Past,* author Roger Ekirch explains that most people divided the night into two five-hour phases: "first sleep" and "second sleep," with a hour or more of wakefulness in between, perhaps to restart the fire for heat, or put the animals back outside. Then came the wonders of electricity, and the world as they knew it changed forever. Artificial light extended the evening hours of work productivity and leisure; both of which altered sleep behaviors during the evening hours.

Before you blame your poor sleep habits on Thomas Edison and his long lasting light bulb, keep in mind that our cultural habits today are as much influenced by Puritanical values (worth equals worth) and capitalism, as the invention of Edison's light bulb. Be that as it may, sleep habits have changed dramatically over the decades and they are changing still (not necessarily for the better), as our lives become so greatly influenced by 21st century technology. Today, sleep experts suggest that eight hours is the golden standard, yet they often confide that some people can subsist comfortably on six hours, while others would do best with the "pre-Edison" 10-hour quota.

Why is it that some people can "sleep like a log" while others toss and turn all night? Why are some people "light sleepers" who awake at the slightest whisper or summer breeze, while others are dead to the world all night? Sleep researchers have been studying various aspects of sleep in earnest for over half a century. What they have found is nothing less than fascinating. While it may look like not much is going on when we sleep, practically lifeless, nothing could be further from the truth. One of the first things that sleep researchers observed was that there are several stages of sleep that are repeated throughout the night. Let's take a closer look.

> Today, sleep experts suggest that eight hours is the golden standard, yet they often confide that some people can subsist comfortably on six hours, while others would do best with the "pre-Edison" 10-hour quota.

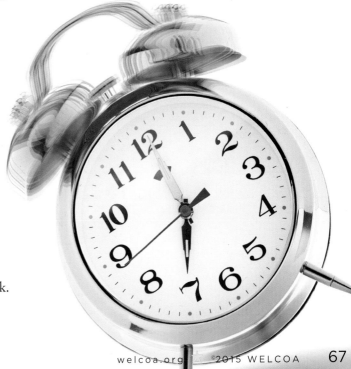

By strategically placing many electrodes on the scalp, neurologists could begin to determine levels of brain activity by the fluctuations (waves) made by electrical signals sent from the electrodes through a transducer to pens on paper.

Sleep Cycles in the Night

Decades ago, experts figured out a way to observe brain activity without any invasive (surgical) means. By strategically placing many electrodes on the scalp, neurologists could begin to determine levels of brain activity by the fluctuations (waves) made by electrical signals sent from the electrodes through a transducer to pens on paper. Electroencephalography (EEG) is the clinical name given to the study of brain waves. A quick review of the variance of brain waves reveals that brain activity becomes important to understand when observing stages of the sleep cycle. These are the five brain wave categories:

Gamma Waves (> 35 Hz)	Extremely active thought processes
Beta Waves (13–30 Hz)	Alertness, mildly active thought processes
Alpha Waves (9–12 Hz)	Relaxed, reflective, contemplative thoughts
Theta Waves (4–8 Hz)	Drowsiness, meditative thoughts
Delta Waves (0.5–3 Hz)	Deep sleep, some dreaming

When the EEG technology was combined with early sleep studies, it became quite evident that there were distinct stages of sleep, based on the fluctuations or patterns of the EEG waves. Moreover, when combined in a linear fashion, the progression of these stages, from Stage 1 to Stage 5 formed what has become known as a "sleep cycle."

Stage 1 Transition Stage (half asleep, half awake) Alpha waves alternate with Theta waves

Stage 2 Alpha waves disappear, Theta waves and spindles, coupled with increased brainwave synchronization

Stage 3 Delta waves and Theta waves

Stage 4 Delta waves (deep sleep)

Stage 5 REM; Rapid Eye Movement (very sound sleep, and dream stage). Fast, irregular brainwaves similar to the waking state. Brain is highly active, but not conscious. In this stage of very deep sleep, dreams, which occur mostly during REM cycles, also appear to be an essential factor for mental equilibrium during the waking hours of a busy day—even if you don't remember them. People who wake before Stage 5 often confide that they didn't sleep very well. Some studies show REM mostly in the last several hours of the night.

Research shows that a complete cycle (Stages 1-5) takes about 90-110 minutes. After the completion of Stage 5, the cycle repeats itself. If you have ever seen movies where someone is sound asleep and there is a loud noise which they sleep right though, but minutes later awaken to the slight sound of a water faucet drip, then you have just seen someone rotate from Stage 5 to Stage 1. People who get less than five to six sleep cycles tend to show signs of sleep deprivation (e.g., general fatigue, poor reaction time, irritability, etc.). Likewise, if someone has several incomplete sleep cycles that miss the REM stage, feelings of fatigue in the waking hours is certain. For this reason it is recommended to have about five to six cycles per night, inclusive of the REM stages. If you do the math, this calculates to about seven to eight hours per night, the recommended quota for each person.

> Not only is the last stage of sleep essential, where dreams unfold, but... the brain's glial cells perform a necessary role in the removal of waste products from the brain's neuron cells.

The Importance of REM

Is one stage of sleep more important than the others? Quite possibly! Sleep experts suggest that the most important stage of the sleep cycle is Stage 5: REM. Here's why: People participating in sleep studies who are repeatedly awoken before this stage occurs show signs of sleep deprivation quite similar to those who cannot fall asleep. Early sleep research revealed that it is the REM period of the sleep cycle where the majority of dreams occur. Although neither EEG nor functional Magnetic Resonant Imaging (fMRI) technology is able to see the actual thoughts/dreams produced during REM, the consensus among sleep researchers is that REM is imperative to cognitive functioning during the waking hours. Additionally, it is interesting to note that not all people get the same amount of REM each night. Infants spend about 50% of their time in REM, whereas healthy adults spend about 20% of sleep in REM each night. REM decreases with the aging process, which may explain why people over the age of 60 claim not to sleep very well, despite sleeping through the night.

The Importance of the Brain's Glial Cells

To say that brain physiology is complicated is no understatement! Not only is the last stage of sleep essential, where dreams unfold, but, as mentioned in Chapter 1, the brain's glial cells perform a necessary role in the removal of waste products from the brain's neuron cells. The human brain is said to be the most complex and dynamic machine in the known universe. While our understanding of it is still quite limited, no doubt many more secrets, like those recently discovered of the brain's glial cells, will be revealed in years to come.

Melatonin: The Zzzz Hormone

Smack in the center of your brain is an organ called the pineal gland. It's small, about the size of a raisin. Its shape and texture resemble that of a pine cone, hence the name pineal (pine-al) gland. In the days of the European Renaissance, René Descartes referred to it as the "seat of the soul." Eastern cultures have also recognized that there is a special part of the brain, "the third eye," associated with intuition, as well as noted divine properties. Today, neurophysiologists stay clear of any metaphysical aspects, but are quite clear in their understanding that the pineal gland produces melatonin; the hormone essential for quality sleep. Current research suggests that the production of melatonin, commonly referred to as the "sleep hormone," requires exposure to rapidly diminishing sunlight followed by darkness, picking up sensory information via the optic nerve. As a side note, the average American, who spends so much of his or her time indoors, typically gets less than 10 minutes of direct sunlight exposure per day, thus throwing off one's circadian rhythm. One current theory suggests lack of direct sunlight may also play a significant role in the search for deep sleep, as lack of sunlight disrupts our natural body clock. The implied message is get outside and enjoy the outdoors. Unless you have dark skin, don't forget the sunblock. Melatonin also plays a role regarding skin's pigmentation via the protein melanin.

One current theory suggests lack of direct sunlight may also play a significant role in the search for deep sleep, as lack of sunlight disrupts our natural body clock. The implied message is get outside and enjoy the outdoors.

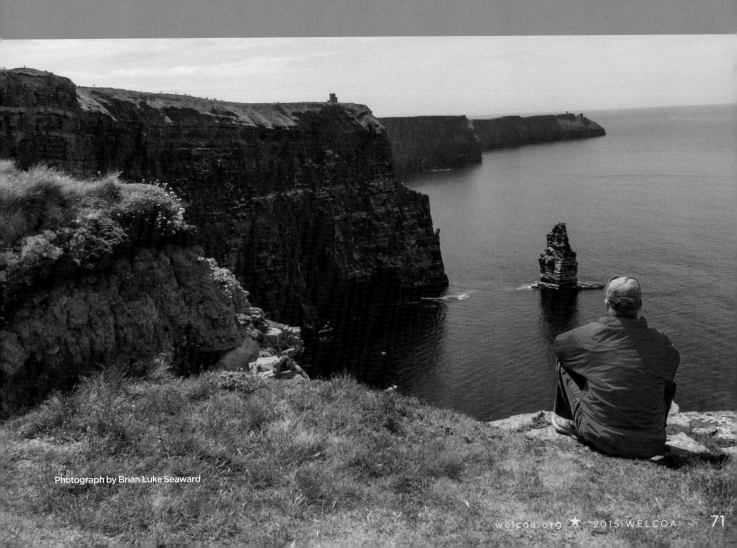

Photograph by Brian Luke Seaward

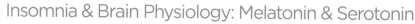

Insomnia & Brain Physiology: Melatonin & Serotonin

As previously stated, brain chemistry is a complicated science and our understanding of it is perhaps embryonic at best. Some facts, however, are clear with regard to how the dynamics of brain physiology works. Not only does an "active" mind release the catacholamines, epinephrine and nor-epinephrine in the brain, compromising the ability to fall sleep, but other neurotransmitters, specifically serotonin, play a role in the sleep hormone equation. Simply stated, the relationship between serotonin and melatonin is crucial in understanding the dynamics of a good night's sleep.

The brain neurotransmitter, serotonin, is partially affected by light as well. Decreases in light decrease serotonin levels, a factor associated with Seasonal Affected Disorder (SAD) and depression. While the use of artificial evening light can alter serotonin levels, it can decrease melatonin levels, thus affecting natural sleep patterns. Increased consumption of carbohydrates (late night snacks) can increase serotonin levels, and this, in turn, may also affect melatonin levels as well. Medications for depression include Selected Serotonin Re-uptake Inhibitor (SSRI) that act to increase serotonin levels, however this may, in fact, act to decrease melatonin levels, thus affecting a full night's sleep. As you can see, brain physiology is quite complex, with many influences both obvious and subtle.

Factors That Decrease Melatonin: A Closer Look

If you like to sleep (and don't we all) then consider melatonin as your best friend. How is your relationship to melatonin? There may be activities and behaviors that are ruining this relationship. Consider this; there are several factors that are known to interrupt the production and secretion of melatonin. As stated above, the exposure to artificial light in the evening hours is thought to have the greatest influence. Artificially warm temperatures also play a key role. Additionally, eating late night snacks consisting of carbohydrates have a significant impact. Carbohydrates increase serotonin levels, hence decreasing melatonin and one's sleep potential. Rounding out this list of melatonin disruptors are medications (mostly those used for depression), the direct light from screen technology (specifically, light in the blue spectrum) and the micro waves from cell phones when held close to the ear, as well as the micro waves from the nearest WiFi router in your house. If you value melatonin, don't take it for granted. Be sure to cultivate a healthy relationship to ensure its highest potential: a good night's sleep.

Types of Insomnia

We have all been there. Lying wide-awake in the dead of night. Nothing, absolutely nothing, it seems, can lull you back into a state of blissful slumber. As polls and medical literature suggest, there are many people who claim to sleep poorly. Some people have a hard time simply falling to sleep. Others (the "light sleepers") may fall asleep easily, but wake up and cannot fall back to sleep. Worrying (stress) about not sleeping, as well as feeling guilty about not sleeping, only exacerbates the problem. Insomnia is a catchall phrase used to describe the lack of sleep, but as one might expect, perhaps from personal experience, there are degrees of poor quality sleep. Through decades of observation and research, sleep experts have categorized the inability to get a good night's sleep into four distinct groups. Let's take a closer look.

1 TRANSIENT INSOMNIA. Transient insomnia (also called acute insomnia) is a term given to people who can sleep well one night and not the next. They may go several nights not being able to sleep at all, perhaps even an entire week. Then, for whatever reason (e.g., resolved stress), they are able to return to a normal sleep cycle. The word transient means something that comes and goes, but doesn't stay very long. Such is the case with transient insomnia. While it may seem quite bothersome, it doesn't last that long.

2 INTERMITTENT INSOMNIA. People who suffer from intermittent insomnia suffer from poor sleep quality for weeks on end. This can be quite frustrating and exhausting.

3 CHRONIC INSOMNIA. The word "chronic" means over a prolonged period of time, and such is the case with chronic insomnia, which lasts months, perhaps even years.

4 REBOUND INSOMNIA. This is a new term in the lexicon of sleep deprivation. Rebound insomnia is a term used to describe someone who tries to get off of sleep medicine, only to find that in doing so, they are not able to sleep without it. Sleep prescriptions alter brain chemistry, often producing a dependence on it for the desired effect.

Additional types of insomnia include "onset insomnia" where people have difficulty falling asleep and "maintenance insomnia," best described as the inability to stay asleep.

Insomnia is a catchall phrase used to describe the lack of sleep, but as one might expect, perhaps from personal experience, there are degrees of poor quality sleep.

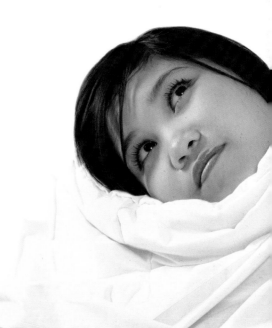

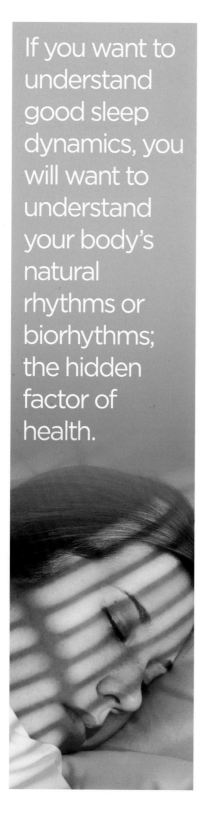

If you want to understand good sleep dynamics, you will want to understand your body's natural rhythms or biorhythms; the hidden factor of health.

A Good Night's Sleep... Ruined

The classification of insomnia (transient, intermittent and chronic) doesn't necessarily address the quantity or quality of sleep in the course of the night, nor does it address the aspects of the sleep cycle itself. For instance, some people may lay awake all night, while others may fall asleep after tossing and turning only to wake up and not be able to fall back asleep. Still, others who fall in the category of "light sleepers" may awaken several times in the course of a night. As you can determine, the anatomy and physiology of a good night's sleep is complicated. One factor to appreciate with sleep is the concept of your body's biorhythms, also known as chronobiology. If you want to understand good sleep dynamics, you will want to understand your body's natural rhythms or biorhythms; the hidden factor of health.

Circadian Rhythms: Calibrating Your Body's Clock

When left to its own devices, unplugged from both high-tech devices and low-tech electrical appliances, the body operates on a 24-hour (circadian) clock. This means that various physiological functions (e.g., hunger, sleep, bowel movements, etc.) fall into a regular and predictable timed sequence. The lack of direct sunlight, the use of artificial light, television, some foods (and food additives) as well as an array of electrical devices are known to throw off these rhythms. When these cycles are derailed, various aspects of health are jeopardized, including gastro-intestinal tract problems, immune function and most notably, sleep patterns. Those who study circadian rhythms as a component of good health suggest that going to bed at the same time every night and waking up at the same time (even on weekends) is ideal to calibrate the body's biological rhythms. But going to bed at a set time each night isn't enough. Several factors must coalesce to form a strong foundation for a good night's sleep, including the foods you eat, the consistent time of each meal, physical activity/exercise and one's bedroom ambiance. So specific are your body's circadian rhythms that oncologists now know that the optimal time for cancer patients to receive chemotherapy is in the early morning hours when DNA repairs are most advantageous. How well-calibrated is your body clock?

The Psychology of Sleep: The Importance of Dreams

It doesn't take a rocket scientist to realize that if psychotic behavior is associated with people who are sleep deprived, then perhaps looking at the mind as well as the brain might be a good idea. However, since the proliferation of psychotropic drug prescriptions by psychiatrists in the 1980s, the field of psychology has focused almost exclusively on the brain and practically ignored the mind, the gateway of the conscience and consciousness.

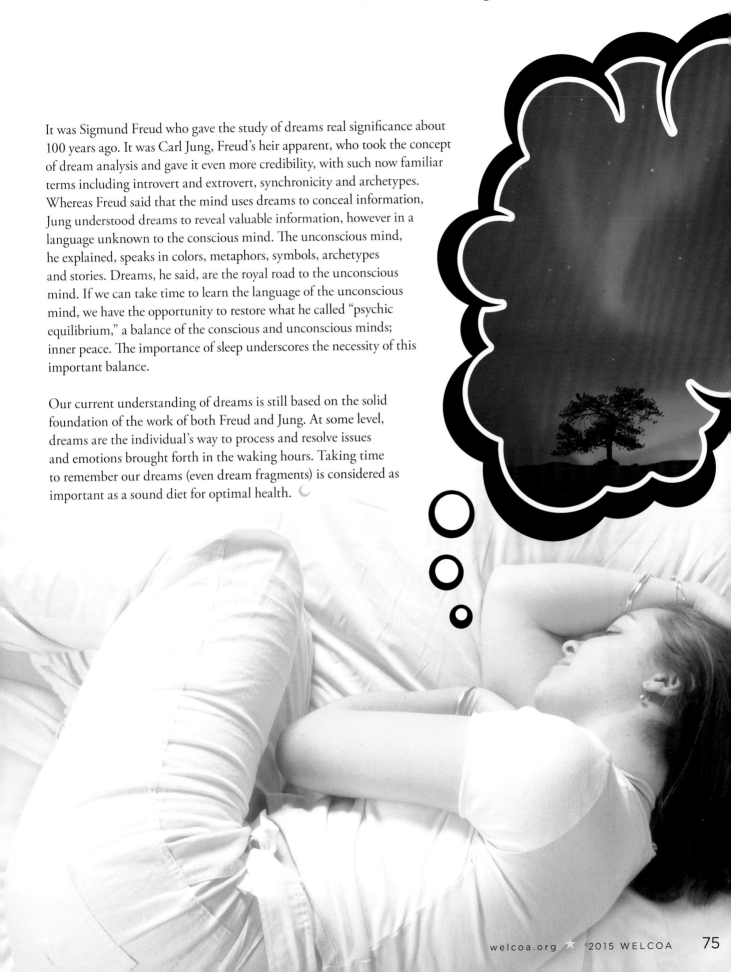

It was Sigmund Freud who gave the study of dreams real significance about 100 years ago. It was Carl Jung, Freud's heir apparent, who took the concept of dream analysis and gave it even more credibility, with such now familiar terms including introvert and extrovert, synchronicity and archetypes. Whereas Freud said that the mind uses dreams to conceal information, Jung understood dreams to reveal valuable information, however in a language unknown to the conscious mind. The unconscious mind, he explained, speaks in colors, metaphors, symbols, archetypes and stories. Dreams, he said, are the royal road to the unconscious mind. If we can take time to learn the language of the unconscious mind, we have the opportunity to restore what he called "psychic equilibrium," a balance of the conscious and unconscious minds; inner peace. The importance of sleep underscores the necessity of this important balance.

Our current understanding of dreams is still based on the solid foundation of the work of both Freud and Jung. At some level, dreams are the individual's way to process and resolve issues and emotions brought forth in the waking hours. Taking time to remember our dreams (even dream fragments) is considered as important as a sound diet for optimal health. ☽

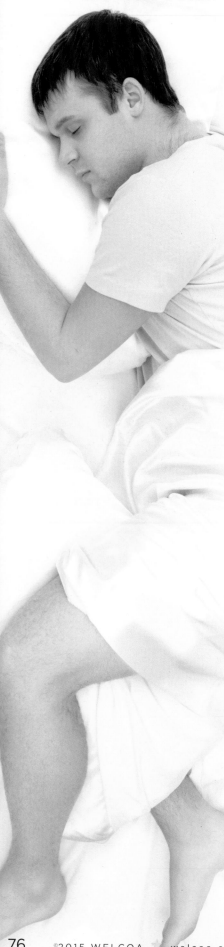

[EXERCISE 4.1]

Dreams Revisited

Although we all have dreams, remembering them is not always easy. But there are occasions when a certain dream is replayed in our mind over the course of months, perhaps even years. Some can even cause us to lose sleep. These recurring dreams may only have a short run on the mind's silver screen (e.g., seconds), or they may last throughout the course of our lifetime. These dreams, perhaps foggy in detail, surface occasionally in the conscious state, and the story they tell is all too familiar. Some issue is begging for resolution.

It is commonly believed that recurring dreams symbolize a hidden insecurity or a stressful event that has yet to be resolved. Simply stated, they don't have resolved endings (e.g., you wake up, sometimes out of sheer panic, before the story in the dream ends). While there is much to the dream state that is still unknown, it is believed that dreams are images that the unconscious mind creates to communicate to the conscious mind in a language all its own. This form of communication is not a one-way street. Messages can be sent to the unconscious mind in a normal waking state as well.

Through the use of mental imagery, you can script the final scenes of a recurring dream with a happy ending. What seems to be the final scene of a dream is actually the beginning of the resolution process. The following is a true story: Once there was a young boy who had an afternoon paper route. One day while the boy was delivering papers, a large black German shepherd jumped out of the bushes and attacked him. The owner called the dog back, but not before the dog drew blood. As the boy grew into adulthood his love for dogs never diminished, but several times a year he awoke in a sweat from a recurring dream he had had once too often. **The Dream:** "It is dark and I am walking through the woods at night. Out from behind one of the trees comes this huge black dog. All I can see are his teeth, and all I can hear is his bark. I try to yell for help, but nothing comes out of my throat. Just as he lunges for me, I awake in a panic."

With a little thought and imagination, a final scene was drafted to bring closure to this dream story. **Final Scene:** "I am walking through the woods at night with a flashlight, a bone, and a can of mace. This time when the dog lunges at me, I shine the light in his eyes and spray mace in his face. He whines and whines, and then I tell him to sit. He obeys. I put the bone by his nose and he looks at me inquisitively. Then he licks the bone and starts to bite into it. I begin to walk away and the dog gets up to follow, bone in mouth. I stop and look back and he stops. He wags his tail. The sky grows light as the sun begins to rise, and the black night fades into pink and orange clouds. As I walk back to my house, I see the dog take his new find down the street. I open the door and walk upstairs and crawl back into bed." It has been five years, and this man has never had this dream again.

Ultimately we are the creators of our dreams. We are the writers, directors, producers, and actors of our dreams. Although drafting a final scene is no guarantee that the issues that produce recurring dreams are resolved, it is a great starting point in the resolution process—a time for reflection that may open up the channels of communication between the conscious and unconscious mind. In fact, in most cases, the active imagination process of completing recurring dreams acts to set things in motion for resolution. Do you have a recurring dream that needs a final scene? Write your recurring dream on the following page and give it a final scene.

The Dream

_____

_____

_____

_____

_____

Final Scene

_____

_____

_____

_____

_____

CHAPTER FIVE

Sleep Robbers

There are some nights when sleep plays coy, aloof and disdainful.

MAYA ANGELOU

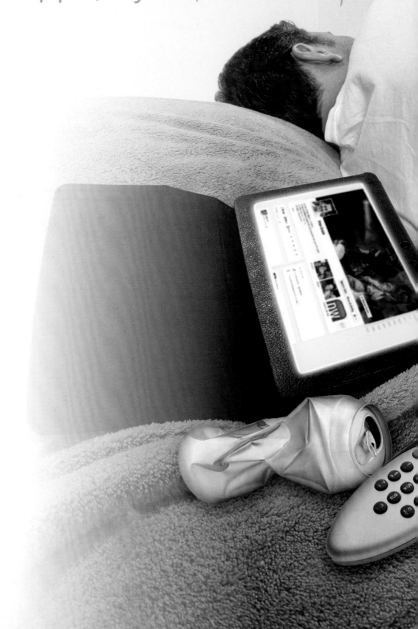

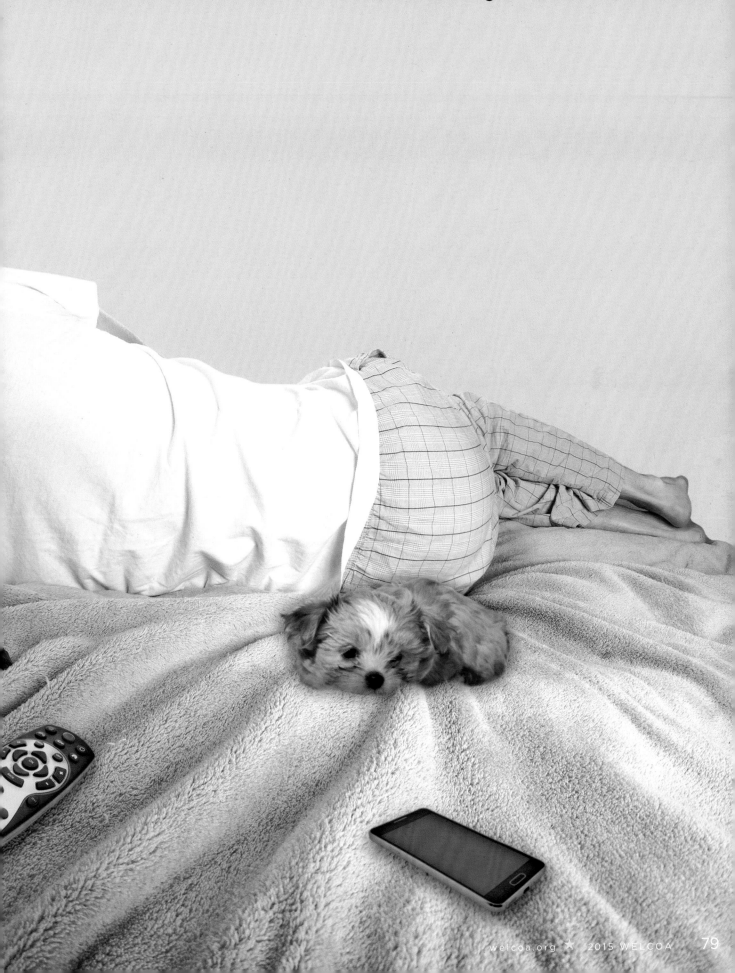

CHAPTER FIVE

Sleep Robbers

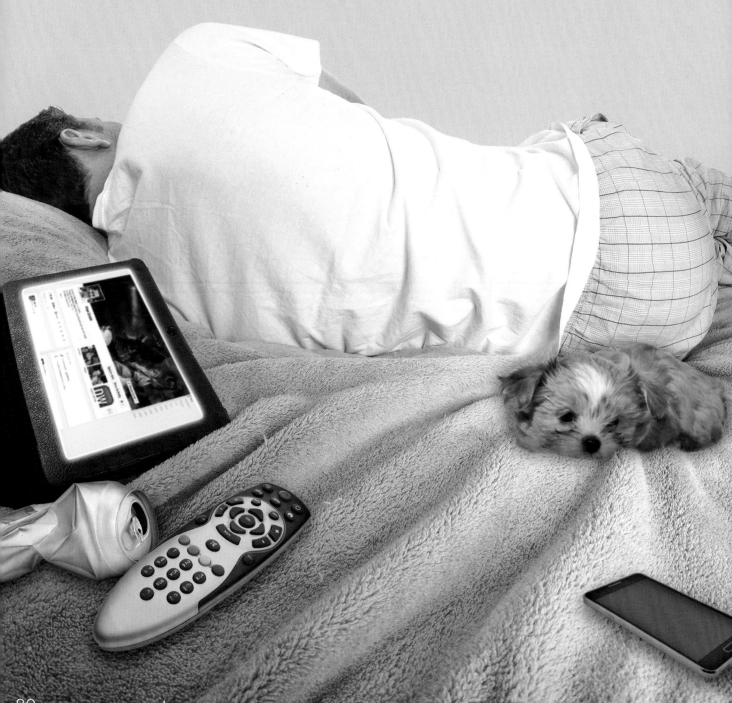

If you were to take a look at Mark's bedroom, you would quickly see why quality of sleep is an issue for him. His bedroom is a mess. Ignoring the carpet of discarded clothes on the floor, his bedroom looks like Captain Kirk's deck of the Starship Enterprise. Between the three monitors on his makeshift home office, the video game console, and the huge flat screen TV, the room is one wall-to-wall liquid crystal display unit. If you stand still and listen quietly, there is a constant hum from all the computers. Moreover, as if entering an Egyptian tomb, the room is guarded by four cats, whose collective purring complements that of the computers. By his bedside, his iPad "pings" repeatedly with each text, email and Facebook update. Because his smart phone has a clever alarm clock app, Mark keeps his cell phone under his pillow when he sleeps (despite the manufacturer's warning NOT to do so). Stated simply, Mark's bedroom is a biohazard; simply not fit for human sleep. A makeover reducing the room to a bed and alarm clock would be a good start. Mark's bedroom is a prime example of poor sleep hygiene; too many distractions in the pursuit of a good night's sleep. It's fair to say that his bedroom is not different than millions of people around the country.

Sleep researchers have a name for the distractions in the bedroom. They call them "sleep robbers." For people who have trouble getting a good night's sleep, sleep robbers serve as major distractions that either delay one from falling asleep (such as watching television or surfing the Internet), or by close proximity simply by their very presence in the bedroom. Indeed, there are many things that can steal a good night's sleep. Remember, we take in information through the portals of our five senses: sight, sound, taste, touch and smell. As we fall into a state of sleep, these portals close one by one. Sleep robbers often enter these portals and as such, it is these same portals that need to be addressed when identifying sleep robbers. Let's take a closer look.

- ☾ **Light.** The ideal sleep environment is one that is completely dark, or pretty close to complete darkness. Light from streetlights, television screens, night-lights, iPads and smart phones, even moonlight can and will be registered by the pineal gland (even with the eyes closed) to affect quality of sleep. Shutting the blinds is a good start. So is sinking deeply into a fluffy down pillow.

- ☾ **Noise.** When the eyes are closed in preparation for sleep, the brain then signals the auditory sense to decrease, similar to turning down, then off, the volume control on the stereo.

Remember, we take in information through the portals of our five senses: sight, sound, taste, touch and smell. As we fall into a state of sleep, these portals close one by one.

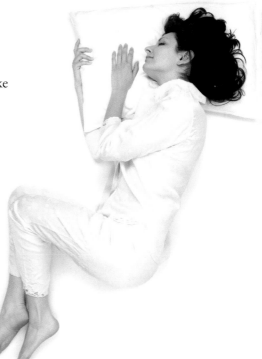

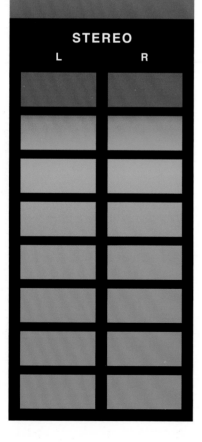

When the eyes are closed in preparation for sleep, the brain then signals the auditory sense to decrease, similar to turning down, then off, the volume control on the stereo.

With a loud noise, however, it can be quickly turned back, as can be verified by people who claim to be light sleepers. Some people choose to sleep with ear plugs as a means to decrease noise and help keep the ports to the sense of sound closed as long as possible.

☽ **Room temperature.** The ideal room temperature for sound sleep is described as cool. Like the Goldielocks approach, it should be neither too cold, nor too hot. The reason for this cool temperature comes back to the regulation of melatonin in the pineal gland that is as much affected by ambient temperature as it is by light. When the bedroom becomes too warm, melatonin production decreases. Some people take a warm shower or bath right before bed, more as a means to relax the muscles than to warm up. If a warm shower or bath works, keep doing it. If, however, you have a hard time falling asleep, cool off a bit after a hot shower before slipping under the covers. If the bedroom is too warm, even hot, the ambient temperature confuses the internal body clock to postpone falling asleep or waking up early. Keep the bedroom cool.

☽ **Technology.** For generations, having a television in the bedroom has become quite common, even a status symbol. However, since the advent of hand-held screen devices, the bedroom has become invaded with technology, all of which serves as a major distraction to quality sleep. In 2012, The National Sleep Foundation issued a statement citing that across America, technology had invaded the bedroom proving to be a formidable force to be reckoned with to ensure a good night's sleep.

☽ **Sleep partner.** Sharing a bed may be great for physical intimacy, but it can be a disaster for a good night's sleep, particularly if your spouse or partner snores loudly, or moves around a lot (e.g., restless leg syndrome). Are separate beds or bedrooms the answer? You will only know by trying it out.

☽ **Pets.** Cats or dogs may be great house pets, but they are not ideal bed companions. Purring, grooming, stretching, shaking and nesting on the bed serves as a distraction, particularly if you are a light sleeper. Cats, more than dogs, can be quite persistent in purposely waking their owners out of a sound sleep. Consider healthy boundaries with your house pets.

If the bedroom is too warm, even hot, the ambient temperature confuses the internal body clock to postpone falling asleep or waking up early. Keep the bedroom cool.

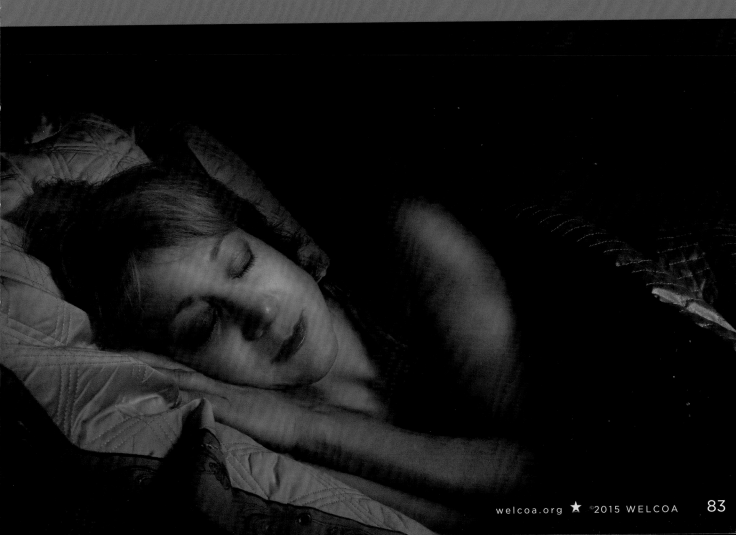

A cluttered bedroom, from clothes on the floor to items lined up against the wall, becomes a metaphor for a cluttered mind; one easily distracted from the purpose at hand, quality sleep. Consider keeping your room clutter-free.

☾ **Caffeine Consumption.** Caffeine is a stimulant. It can be found in coffee, tea, chocolate and many types of sodas. People consume caffeine as a means to wake up or perk up. Caffeine acts on the sympathetic nervous system by releasing epinephrine and nor-epinephrine; the stress catecholamine. When the brain is engaged in the stress response via caffeine, the ability to fall asleep and stay asleep is greatly compromised. Remember, it takes eight hours to metabolize one 8-ounce cup of coffee. Knowing this, it would make good sense not to consume foods and beverages that contain caffeine if you have troubles sleeping.

☾ **Clutter.** A cluttered bedroom, from clothes on the floor to items lined up against the wall, becomes a metaphor for a cluttered mind; one easily distracted from the purpose at hand, quality sleep. Consider keeping your room clutter-free.

Sleep robbers don't just include how your bedroom looks or even your behavior right before bed. They also include behaviors you engage in well before bedtime; from food and beverages you consume during the course of a day to the moment you walk into your house after an 8-10 hour workday. Here are some other aspects to keep in mind that sow the seeds for sleep robbers to steal your precious sleep.

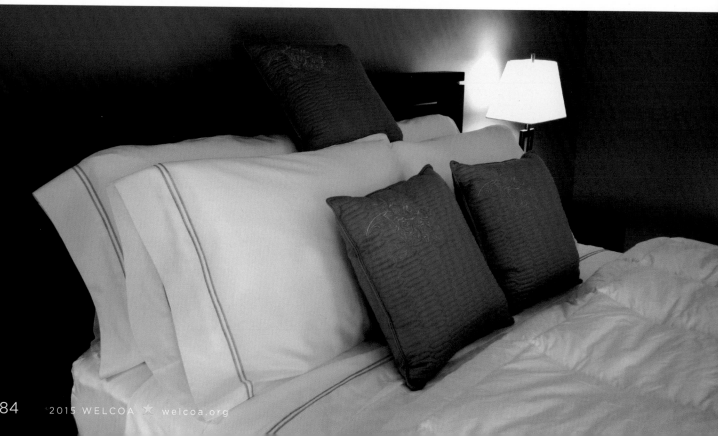

Foods, Acid Reflux and Disturbed Sleep

Many people today suffer from a condition known as acid reflux (also called heartburn or simply indigestion) where stomach acids that digest food begin to backflow up into the esophagus. Not only does this taste horrible, but if you accidentally breathe this into your lungs, it can cause serious health problems. People who suffer from acid reflux wake up an hour or so after falling asleep choking on these stomach acids. Not only does acid reflux disturb you out of a sound sleep, but repeated episodes can prevent you from falling back asleep. If you have ever wondered why people drink a glass of milk before bed, this is the reason. The alkalinity of milk is thought to reduce the acid build up in the stomach.

Heartburn, as a physical malady, has been around for eons, but the prevalence of it has increased dramatically in the past decade. What causes acid reflux? Anatomically speaking, the valve that closes the esophagus to food becomes floppy with age, thus allowing for a backwash of stomach acid when you are in the prone (sleeping) position. The common advice for acid reflux includes the following:

☾ Eat dinner at least four hours before bedtime.

☾ Chew your food before swallowing it. The recommended number of times to chew your food is 30 times. Most people chew once, if that, and swallow, giving rise to the expression "wolfing" your food down. Chew slowly and chew often.

☾ Some foods are more conducive to acid reflux than others. For this reason these types of foods are not recommended to include as a part of your evening meal. These foods include: red meats, tomatoes, coffee and tea, carbonated drinks, spices (often found in Chinese, Indian and Mexican foods) as well as garlic and onions.

☾ Health food stores sell natural herbal remedies for acid reflux that have no side effects when consumed.

When things move fast on a TV screen, so much so that you cannot take your eyes off it, you are engaged in a low-level stress response. When you are engaged in the stress response you are not relaxed!

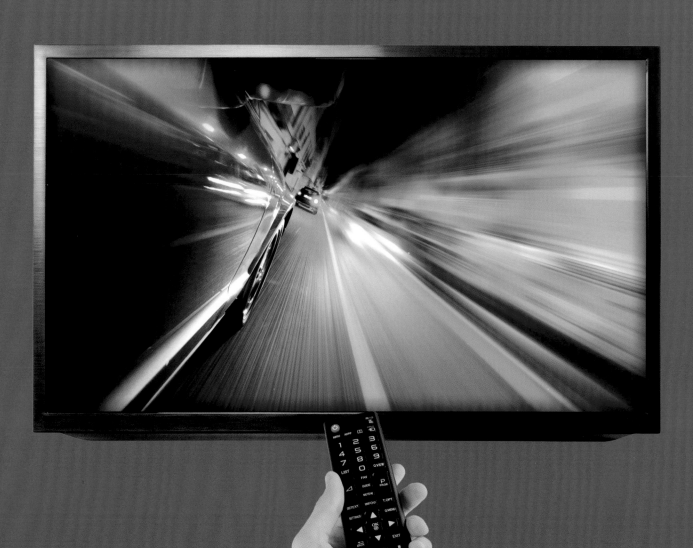

Excuse Me, TV Viewing Is Not Relaxing

Many people sit down and watch several hours of television before they turn in for the night. In fact, this behavior has become a national pastime. "Vegging out" in front of the television, they claim, is "relaxing." While sitting with your legs up on the coffee table may look (even feel) relaxing, engaging your brain with what is on the flat screen TV is not really relaxing. Here is why:

Before the invention of the remote control, people had to get up out of their chairs and walk across the living room to change the channel. With a remote control in hand, changing the channel could happen immediately, without moving more than a few muscles in the hand. Advertisers were the first to notice that the television viewing public was skipping the ads, ads that paid for the television programming. So television producers were forced to change the production of filming television shows, even theater movies to keep the viewer lured in with their eyes glued to the screen.

Have you ever noticed that scenes on television shows change very quickly and dialogue between characters is brief (no soliloquies)? There is a legitimate reason for this. Advertising marketing executives caught on long ago that if things moved really quickly on the television screen, it kept your attention, which is exactly what they want to do. Between the movement of actors, camera motion, the quick pace of camera angles, and split-second editing, television shows today seem to be hyped up with fast paced movement, all to keep you engaged.

If you have ever watched old movies and television shows filmed before 1985, you may have thought to yourself, gee the action seems rather slow, perhaps even boring. To a brain that has been trained to view fast-action editing, indeed, older shows are much slower-paced. By comparison, today's viewing selection is much more riveting, engaging and exciting.

How does watching TV today become stressful? When scenes or actions move fast on a TV screen, so much so that you cannot take your eyes off it, you are engaged in a low-level stress response. When you are engaged in the stress response you are not relaxed! When this aspect of television is combined with the content (e.g., storylines built on tension and violence), the overall effect is anything but relaxing. It takes longer to calm the mind after watching hours of television which is why watching television in bed is not ideal.

Does this mean you should not watch television before bed? We will leave this up to you. But, if you have a hard time falling asleep at night with a mind that races all over the place, this might be something to consider more seriously.

> Between the movement of actors, camera motion, the quick pace of camera angles, and split-second editing, television shows today seem to be hyped up with fast paced movement, all to keep you engaged.

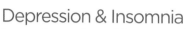

Depression & Insomnia

Insomnia may be problematic in the United States, but depression is even more so. Current estimates suggest that four billion prescriptions for anti-depressants are written each year. How are depression and insomnia related? The answer is complicated, but here is a brief synopsis. Neurophysiology studies regarding the complex topic of brain chemistry reveal that depression is associated with a decrease in the production of the neuropeptide, serotonin. Serotonin is often referred to as the "happy hormone." High (normal) amounts make you feel good; low amounts can make you feel depressed.

As natural sunlight decreases at the end of each day and ambient temperature drops, the body's circadian rhythms send a signal to the pineal gland (the pine cone-shaped organ in the center of the brain) to start making melatonin. As melatonin increases, serotonin decreases (some neurophysiologists suggest that the formation of melatonin comes from the chemical breakdown of serotonin). As melatonin increases, the urge to sleep increases and off to bed we go. Problems arise when people who are diagnosed as being clinically depressed are taking medications (usually selective serotonin reuptake inhibitor, SSRI's) to keep serotonin levels elevated. Hence, in an effort to keep serotonin levels high, efforts to synthesize and release melatonin are greatly diminished. Consequently people who are on medications have a hard time falling asleep because of the melatonin/serotonin imbalance. If they take a prescription to sleep, the delicate balance of brain chemistry is thrown off even more, complicating an already complicated situation.

Afternoon Naps: Good or Bad?

To curl up on a sofa under a warm blanket and close your eyes for just a few moments sounds heavenly. And it is. To lay outstretched on your king-size bed and sink into the nest of down pillows on a Sunday afternoon sounds delightful. And it is.

But sleep researchers warn that taking naps in the daylight hours may throw off one's circadian rhythms, thus interrupting a good night's sleep. While some people warn against a short afternoon nap, other health experts see naps as a good thing, honoring the body's desire to rest. You know what works best for you. If you love afternoon naps, but find that you cannot sleep through the night the same night, then naps may not be the best option for you. ☾

[EXERCISE 5.1]

Sleep Robber Checklist

The following is a simple checklist to critique your sleep ambiance and help you determine to what extent good quality sleep is being robbed from you. On a scale of 1-5 (1 = very poor, 5 = excellent), please rate your sleep environment based on these factors. Anything less than good can be a red flag.

RATING:	EXCELLENT	GOOD	FAIR	POOR	VERY POOR
1. Light/darkness factor	5	4	3	2	1
2. Noise factor	5	4	3	2	1
3. Temperature factor	5	4	3	2	1
4. Bedding factor	5	4	3	2	1
5. Routine/ritual	5	4	3	2	1
6. Technology (iPad, mobile phone)	5	4	3	2	1
7. Television in bedroom	5	4	3	2	1
8. TV watching before sleep	5	4	3	2	1
9. Meals close to bedtime	5	4	3	2	1
10. Sleeping partner	5	4	3	2	1
11. Pets	5	4	3	2	1
12. Caffeine intake before bed	5	4	3	2	1
13. Chronic pain	5	4	3	2	1
14. Medications	5	4	3	2	1
15. Naps during the day	5	4	3	2	1
16. Other _____	5	4	3	2	1

Key: If you scored more than eight items as fair or lower, then it's time to take a closer look at your sleep ambiance and sleep hygiene habits.

Based on this quick survey, what changes can you make to your sleep environment?

_____

_____

_____

_____

_____

_____

CHAPTER SIX

Good Zzzzzzleep Management

A good laugh and a long sleep are the best cures for anything.

IRISH PROVERB

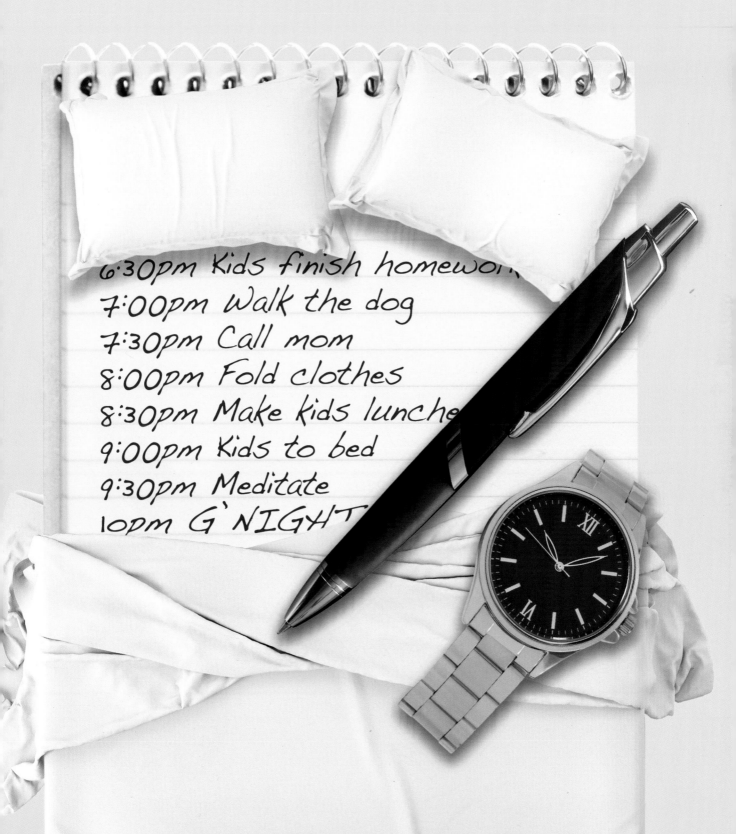

6:30pm Kids finish homework
7:00pm Walk the dog
7:30pm Call mom
8:00pm Fold clothes
8:30pm Make kids lunches
9:00pm Kids to bed
9:30pm Meditate
10pm G'NIGHT!

CHAPTER SIX

Good Zzzzzzleep Management

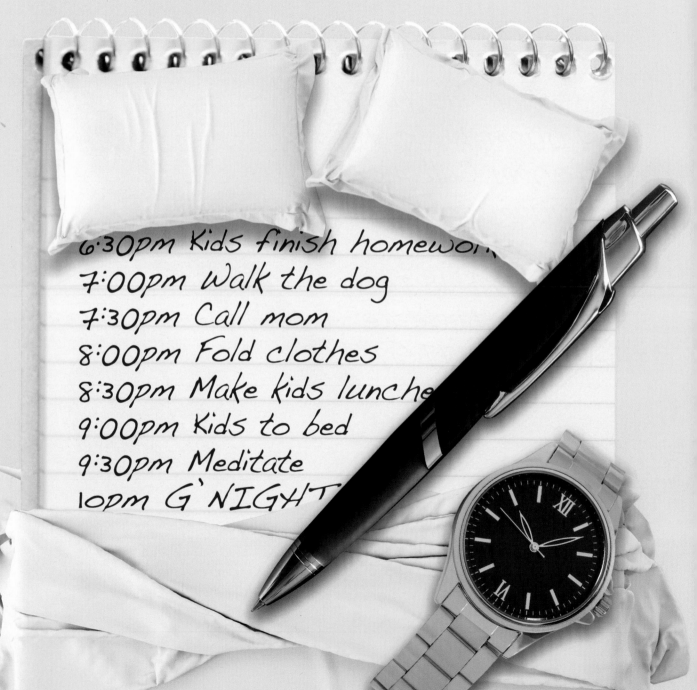

6:30pm Kids finish homework
7:00pm Walk the dog
7:30pm Call mom
8:00pm Fold clothes
8:30pm Make kids lunches
9:00pm Kids to bed
9:30pm Meditate
10pm G'NIGHT!

Sean has a routine before he goes to bed to ensure a good night's sleep. His evening ritual is a calculated strategy to allow his mind and body to unwind well before he climbs into bed. His routine begins at 8:30 p.m. with making a cup of herbal (chamomile) tea. As the pot of water starts to boil, he lets the dog out in the backyard to do his business. Once the dog is back inside, as the tea steeps in the porcelain mug, Sean checks the locks on all the doors and turns the heat off. With a hot cup of tea in hand, he sits on the living room sofa, with some soft instrumental guitar music playing on the stereo. With a pad of paper and pen, he makes his "to do" list for the next day. Alongside of this list, he makes a list of the highlights of the present day. Then, for a few moments, he closes his eyes and focuses on his breathing; "mindfulness breathing" he calls it. Sometimes he may read a book for 30 minutes or quietly listen to more music. At 9:45 p.m., before he walks into the bedroom, he enters the home office, places his smart phone on the desk, turns off all computers (laptop, desktop and iPad), and the WiFi router. Then all remaining lights in the house go off, save the bedroom and bathroom. With toothpaste on his brush, then dental floss, his teeth get a devotional period of attention. After a few additional responsibilities in the bathroom, the alarm clock is checked for a 5:30 a.m. wake-up. With the bedroom lights off at 10:00 p.m. and the window shades drawn closed, Sean crawls into bed laying on soft Egyptian cotton sheets (800 thread count), lays his head on the down pillow and is fast asleep, next to his wife, who is already fast asleep.

Whether you sleep like a rock or not, sleep experts say it is ideal to have a bedtime routine (some call it a ritual) every night, and to be consistent with it. People who have a hard time sleeping often have a minimal routine at best, with many behaviors that sabotage sound sleep. The purpose of a good pre-bedtime routine is to program your evening behaviors with a relaxation strategy that allows your mind to calm down, as a way to "enter the realm" of quality sleep. Remember, having an evening ritual is only as good as the follow-through to make it happen. Proper discipline is important. Like any skill, repetition (practice) over a couple of week's time allows it to become second nature (Exercise 6.1 invites you to fine-tune your pre-sleep routine).

The purpose of a good pre-bedtime routine is to program your evening behaviors with a relaxation strategy that allows your mind to calm down, as a way to "enter the realm" of quality sleep.

All aspects of good sleep hygiene require the recognition and enforcement of healthy boundaries to promote a good night's sleep consistently.

The Essence of Good Sleep Hygiene: A Review

Let's revisit some sleep basics: Experts in the field of sleep wellness refer to an ideal sleep environment as good "sleep hygiene." Like the importance of personal hygiene (e.g., brushing one's teeth, taking a daily shower, having clean underwear, etc.), sleep hygiene is equally essential for personal health and wellness. One might think that creating a quality sleep environment is nothing less than obvious, but this is not always the case. Many personal behaviors and bedrooms across America are anything but conducive for promoting a consistent good night's sleep.

Stress plays a big role in the quality of sleep (or lack thereof), but there are many other aspects that contribute to what sleep experts call "sleep hygiene;" also known as the ambiance of your bedroom. For example, as explained in the previous chapter, room temperature plays a big role in the quality of sleep. Core body temperature drops in the evening hours as the body prepares to shut down in sleep mode. A room with an elevated temperature doesn't allow one's body core temp to do its job (note: this may explain the relationship between menopausal hot flashes and poor sleep quality). Secondly, good sleep hygiene requires darkness. Night-lights, bright alarm clock lights, even the full moon radiance as well as outside streetlights are all registered by the pineal gland, even when your eyes are shut, and this will affect the production and secretion of melatonin. Noise will certainly affect the quality of one's sleep hygiene as well. Noises include everything from your partner's snoring or teeth grinding (note: TMJ is a sign of latent anger) to a blaring television, as well as the house pet's self-grooming on the bed or ambulance sirens. Any disturbance to the five senses that impedes quality sleep is called "sleep robbers." All aspects of good sleep hygiene require the recognition and enforcement of healthy boundaries to promote a good night's sleep consistently.

Core body temperature drops in the evening hours as the body prepares to shut down in sleep mode. A room with an elevated temperature doesn't allow one's body core temp to do its job…

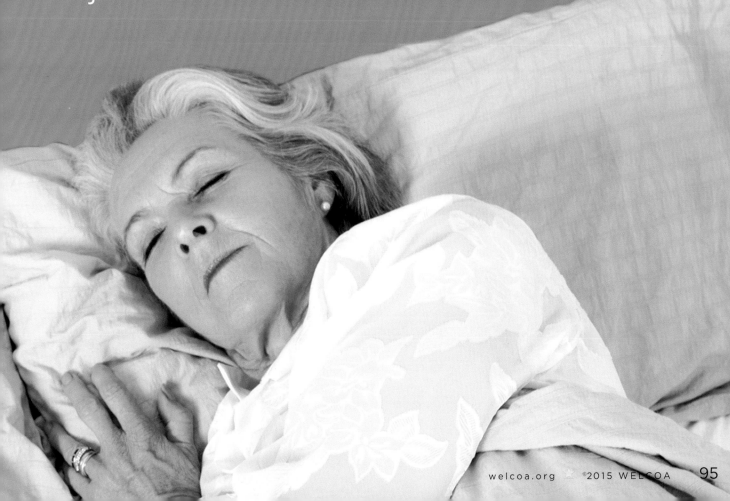

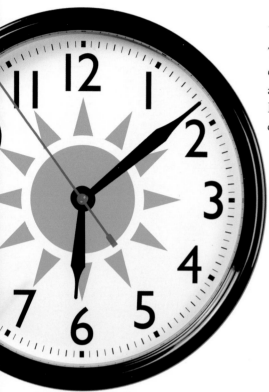

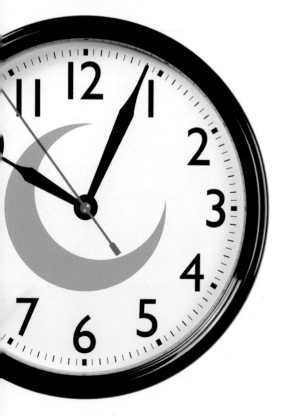

Tips to Improve Your Sleep Hygiene

The following is a quick checklist to help you promote a healthier sleep environment. When reviewing your personal checklist, consider paying attention to these five senses: sight, sound, taste, touch and smell. Remember, first and foremost, bedrooms are for sleeping, and not much else. As you survey your bedroom, first consider what to subtract/remove.

1 KEEP A REGULAR SLEEP CYCLE. Make a habit of going to bed at the same time every night (within 15 minutes) and waking up about the same time each morning (even on weekends). You also might consider honoring your circadian rhythms by eating your dinner at approximately the same time each night as well. Many sleep experts note that one should not eat a big meal right before falling asleep, as the digestion process will interfere with one's sleep cycles (REM). Remember to honor your biorhythms.

2 INSTITUTE A DIGITAL CURFEW. Back in the days before cell phones, most teenagers heard their parents invoke this household rule: no phone calls after 9:00 p.m. Given the problems with cell phones and the production of melatonin, not to mention screen addictions and the incessant lure of social networking, invoking a digital curfew is an excellent idea to promote. Having a digital curfew means that all things digital get turned off at least an hour before bedtime.

3 CREATE YOUR IDEAL SLEEP AMBIANCE. Your bedroom is your sleep sanctuary. As such, it is essential to create a sleep-friendly environment where bright lights, noise and all other sensory distractions are minimized, if not completely eliminated. Additionally, invest in a good quality comfortable bed and bedding (e.g., high thread count sheets, down pillows and comforters). For a place in which you spend one-third of your life, consider the best options to promote quality sleep. You deserve the best. Remember, there is a good reason why the exclusive hotels around the world furnish their first class beds with Italian or Egyptian cotton sheets, down pillows and comforters. Start with a good mattress, but don't end there. Continue with a superior mattress pad, the highest quality sheets (higher thread counts equals a softness that lulls you into la-la land), and goose down pillows. Think of your bed as the throne of the castle, not the dungeon.

A   LIGHT/DARKNESS AMBIANCE. Be sure to cover all windows with shades or thick curtains to ensure a dark ambiance. Also, rather than leaving a light on in the bathroom, consider installing a motion sensor light that only comes on when you need it. Night-lights will affect your pineal gland and sabotage the work of melatonin.

B   ROOM TEMPERATURE. As evening ambient temperature decreases, this signals to the pineal gland to increase the secretion of melatonin. If your bedroom is warm or uncomfortably warm, this may interrupt your sleep quality. Some people prefer an open window with fresh air to a stuffy hot room.

C   PETS. There is a popular cartoon on YouTube where a cat does everything to wake up Simon, his caretaker. When nothing works, he pulls out a baseball bat from behind the bed and slams the guy in the head, then innocently curls up at the foot of the bed. It's funny, and as all cat owners know, all too real. Pets may be members of your family, but having cats and dogs on your bed while you sleep can be a huge distraction. First, as any pet owner knows, cats and dogs have different sleep cycles than their human housemates. Moreover, self-grooming pets can wake you out of a sound sleep. Establish healthy boundaries and keep pets out of the bedroom. Good luck and keep all bats out of the bedroom!

D   CREATE A TECH-FREE BEDROOM (NO SCREEN GADGETS). Simply stated, technology does not belong in the bedroom. Make your bedroom a tech-free zone. Computers, tablets, cell phones and televisions should be removed. Seriously consider unplugging the WiFi router before you go to bed as well (WiFi micro waves negatively affect the pineal gland). Electric alarm clocks should be more than five feet from your head when you sleep.

E   SLEEPING COMFORT. If you spend a third of your life sleeping, make it comfortable. This includes high thread count sheets (we strongly consider 750 or higher), down pillows and a down comforter. A good mattress pad is also suggested. Down pillows

> If your bedroom is warm or uncomfortably warm, this may interrupt your sleep quality. Some people prefer an open window with fresh air to a stuffy hot room.

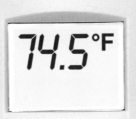

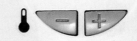

If noise is a problem consider some type of white noise to balance out the distracting sounds that impede your quality of sleep. Listening to soft music (preferably instrumental music) may help you fall asleep as well.

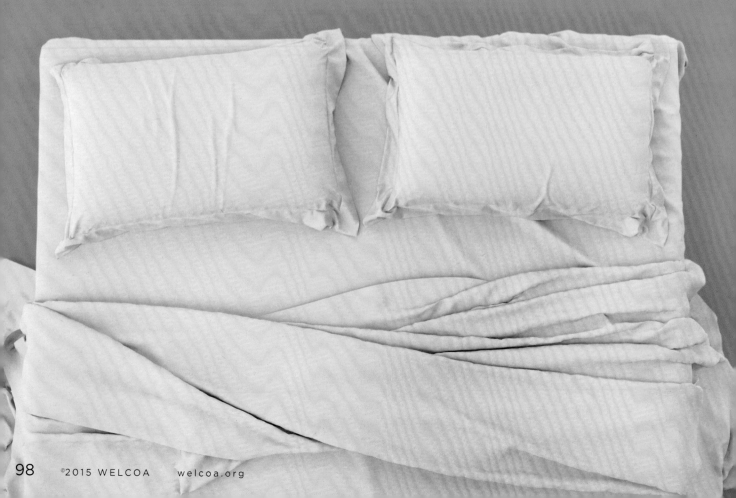

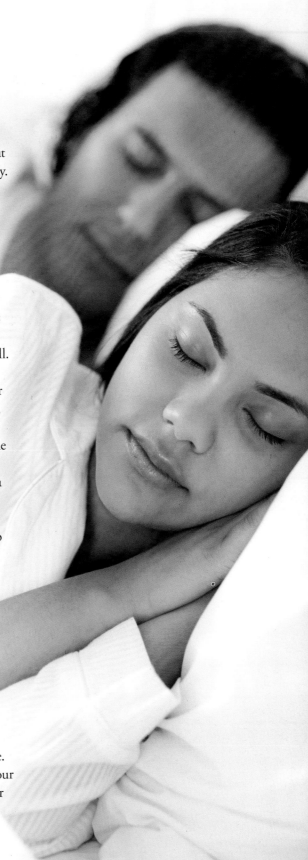

can be washed or dry-cleaned, and should be cleaned regularly. Note that foam rubber pillows cannot be washed. Flipping the mattress every three to four months is a good idea as well. Sleeping comfort may also include the clothes you sleep in. We recommend no electronics associated with the bed as well. Depending on the make, the life span of a good mattress is about 10-15 years. Be sure to rotate and turn over the mattress regularly.

F   A QUIET BEDROOM: NOISE REDUCTION. Needless to say, your bedroom should be quiet but certain noises may prevent total silence, from police sirens to your spouse snoring. While you cannot control all distracting sounds, you can balance them with white noise (e.g., podcasts of ocean waves, waterfalls, etc.). If noise is a problem, consider some type of white noise to balance out the distracting sounds that impede your quality of sleep. Listening to soft music (preferably instrumental music) may help you fall asleep as well.

G   SLEEP PARTNERS. Sleeping with a spouse or partner may be very comforting, but it may also have some limitations, particularly if the person you share the bed with snores loudly, or has restless leg syndrome (RLS) where sudden motions of the arms or legs may awake you. Evaluate your bed partner. It may be that sleeping in separate beds is the only solution to a good night's sleep.

H   FOOD AND SNACKS. While some people may keep a snack nearby, experts agree that the bedroom is for sleeping and it is the one room in the house where food and snacks should not be eaten (unless you are bedridden with an illness). Food often serves as a distraction and as such, it is best to honor the concept of healthy boundaries and keep all food out of the bedroom. A glass of water (or water bottle) on the other hand is encouraged.

I   OTHER DISTRACTIONS. There are countless distractions that can interrupt a good night's sleep, including behaviors hours before bedtime. Only you know what these are. By making note of these and including beneficial changes in your pre-sleep routine you begin to create a solid foundation for your sleep wellness.

The bottom line is that exercise, specifically cardiovascular exercise, is essential for quality sleep.

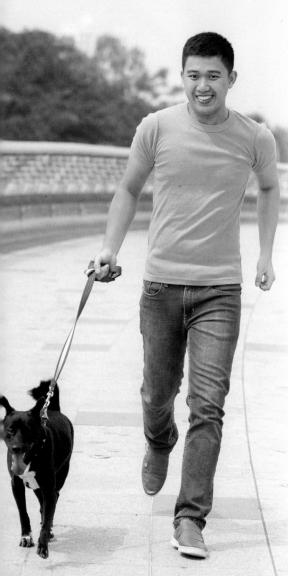

4 GET OUT AND EXERCISE. Daily cardiovascular exercise such as walking, swimming, jogging or cycling acts to reset one's physiology for optimal balance by flushing out stress hormones (e.g., cortisol, aldosterone and vasopressin) produced and secreted in the course of a hectic day. In the course of physical exercise, you flush these hormones out of the body, ensuring a better senses of homeostasis. The bottom line is that exercise, specifically cardiovascular exercise, is essential for quality sleep. Consider a daily 20-30 minute walk before dinner. Exercise after dinner, before bed is not recommended.

5 DECREASE YOUR CAFFEINE CONSUMPTION. Caffeine is a stimulant, and the most popular drug in the world. Remember, it takes eight hours to metabolize one (1) 8-ounce cup of coffee. If you are trying to relax, a neurological stimulant is the last thing you want to put into your body. Coffee, tea and soft drinks are a poor choice of beverage if you have problems sleeping. Consider avoiding drinking any beverages with caffeine (coffee, tea, sodas, even chocolate) after 6:00 p.m. as the effects of caffeine on the nervous system promote a stress response (arousal) rather than a relaxation effect (sleep). Herbal teas are a great alternative, as is filtered water with a slice of lemon.

6 LEARN TO MEDITATE. Meditation is a simple practice to discipline the mind for clear thinking. The best definition I have come across for meditation is "increased concentration that leads to increased awareness." Meditation can be as simple as 1) finding a comfortable spot to sit quietly, 2) closing your eyes, and 3) focusing entirely on your breathing. When interrupting thoughts enter your mind, let them go as you exhale. Start with sitting still for five minutes and work your way up to 15 minutes over a few weeks. People who meditate not only sleep better in the evening; they are more grounded and present in the waking hours (Chapter 7 highlights the aspect of mindfulness meditation).

7 THROW OUT YOUR TV. Avoid watching television right before you go to bed. Instead, try reading to induce a sense of drowsiness. If your television is in your bedroom, move it out. If your children have a TV in their bedroom, do the same. If you cannot bear to throw out your television, create healthy boundaries with your TV habits. Remember, the TV does not belong in the bedroom.

8 AVOID ALCOHOL AND NICOTINE. Constituents found in both alcohol and nicotine excite the central nervous system thus causing a disturbance in brain chemistry required for a good night's sleep (by the way, milk contains the neuropeptide tryptophan which is known to help induce sleep).

9 CLEAR YOUR LATE NIGHT MIND. Make a to-do list right before you go to bed to cleanse your mind of racing thoughts. Keep the pad of paper by your bed in the event you think of more things as your head hits the pillow. By placing items and responsibilities on paper you won't be as inclined to obsess about them during coveted sleep hours.

10 YOUR BED IS FOR SLEEPING. In this 24/7 society, beds have become second home offices (e.g., balancing checkbooks, grading papers, reviewing taxes, etc.) Beds have also become recliners for watching TV and even a second dinner table. Good sleeping requires healthy boundaries. In this case remove all non-sleep activities from your bedroom. Keep your bed as a vehicle for sleep (and sex) and leave it at that. ☾

Keep a pad of paper by your bed in the event you think of more things as your head hits the pillow.

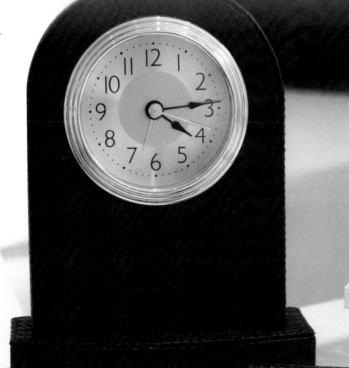

The purpose of a good pre-bedtime routine is to program your evening behaviors with a relaxation strategy that allows your mind to calm down, as a way to "enter the realm" of quality sleep.

[EXERCISE 6.1]

Fine-Tuning Your Pre-Sleep Routine

What does your nighttime routine look like? Do you even have one? What do you do to prepare for a good night's sleep? Honestly, how is your sleep hygiene? If you have a hard time sleeping and your answer is nothing more than turning out the lights and crawling into bed, you might consider taking some time to chart your evening activities before you call it a night. What time do you turn off your tablet or smart phone and wifi router? What time do you brush your teeth? What do you do in the evening hours and are there any things to change to promote a better night's sleep for you? So, what does your pre-sleep routine look like? Start with what you do immediately after dinner. Conclude with surveying any intentions while you lay your head on the pillow to sleep, (e.g., remember your dreams, finding solutions to problems, etc.). Start by making a chronological list in 15-minute increments with the goal to be in bed by 10:00 p.m.

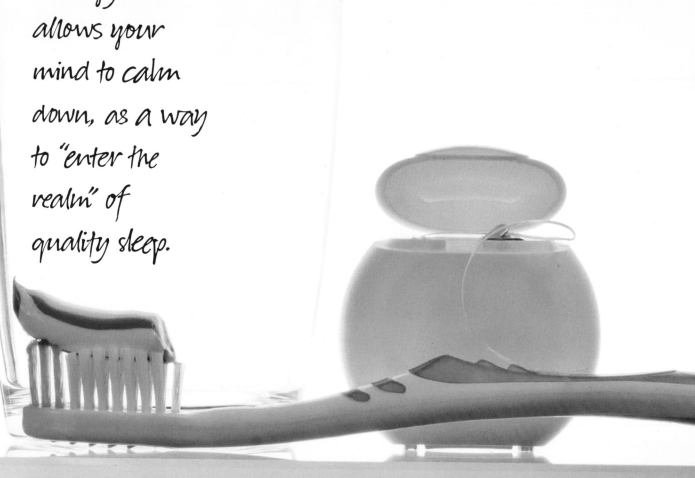

Your Pre-Sleep Routine

7:30 p.m. _____

_____

7:45 p.m. _____

_____

8:00 p.m. _____

_____

8:15 p.m. _____

_____

8:30 p.m. _____

_____

8:45 p.m. _____

_____

9:00 p.m. _____

_____

9:15 p.m. _____

_____

9:30 p.m. _____

_____

9:45 p.m. _____

_____

10:00 p.m. _____

_____

10:05 p.m. _Crawl into bed, snug under the covers._

Zzzzzzzzz...

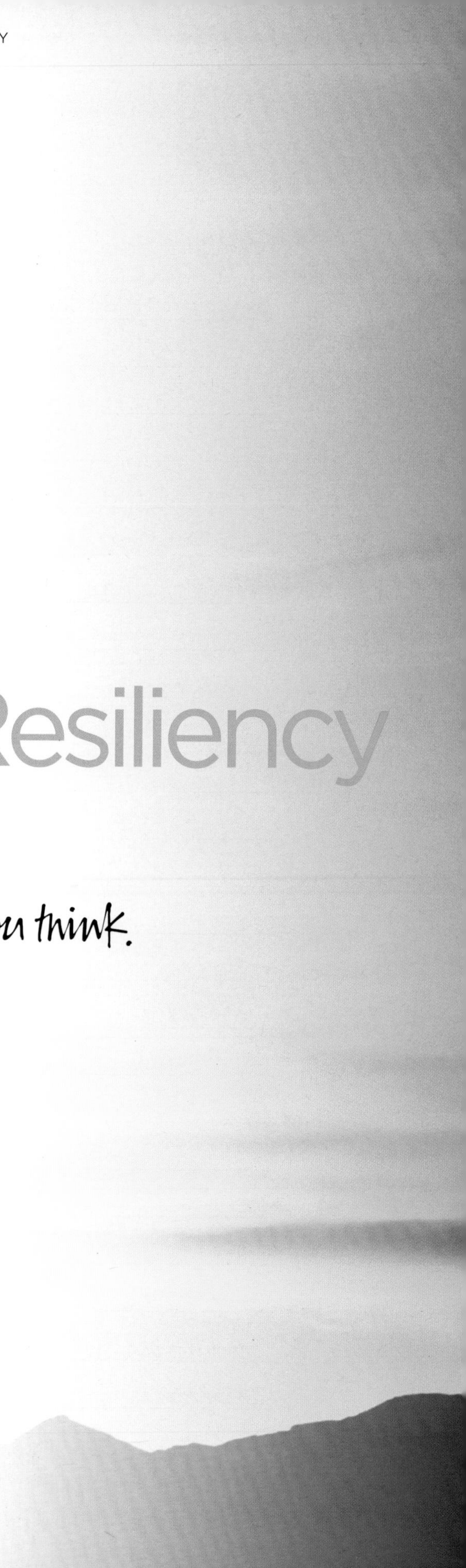

CHAPTER SEVEN

Mindfulness Resiliency

Meditation; It's not what you think.

ANONYMOUS

Photograph by Brian Luke Seaward

CHAPTER SEVEN

Mindfulness Resiliency

If you feel like the pace of life has picked up dramatically in the past several years, and you feel a bit overwhelmed, not only by the changes, but also the rate of these changes, welcome to the club! Terms like "sensory bombardment," "sensory overload," "monkey-mind" and "burnout" are not new to the American vernacular, but they seem to be used with greater and greater frequency as people navigate their lives through an ever-expanding maze of change. Perhaps one of the biggest changes has been the rapid introduction of hand-held devices, such as smart phones and iPads, that bring the world instantly to your fingertips. When you combine the following aspects: 24/7 lifestyle, instant gratification, voyeurism, multi-tasking, rapid change, and instability in the 21ˢᵗ century lifestyle, it's not hard to grasp the concepts of "sensory bombardment" and "mental burnout." Moreover, we live in a culture of distractions with countless people (and things) begging for our attention. When our attention is divided in several directions and our thoughts are scattered, chronic stress is not far behind.

Enter the age of mindfulness. Mindfulness is a timeless concept associated with the ability to harness the powers of concentration, mental clarity and insight. Simply stated, mindfulness is a focused mind. Although the word mindfulness is often associated with Buddhism, it predates all religions, even meditative practices that claim it as their own. For decades, Olympic athletes referred to mindfulness simply as "mental training." First made popular in the U.S. by Vietnam peace activist, Thich Nhat Hanh several decades ago, and again more recently by stress management expert, Jon Kabat Zinn, mindfulness is a simple type of meditation to gain and maintain mental clarity by living in the moment.

The newest research in mind-body science from the University of Wisconsin-Madison reveals that meditation, specifically mindfulness meditation, has the unique ability to create new neuron cells that can help facilitate better brain function. It's called neuroplasticy.

> When our attention is divided in several directions and our thoughts are scattered, chronic stress is not far behind.

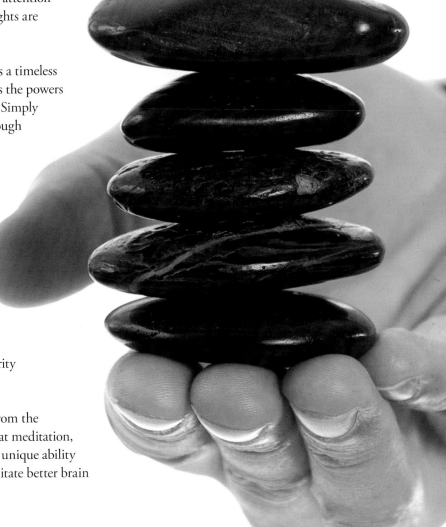

> Neuro-plasticity refers to the brain's ability to restructure itself after periods of training or practice...

Neuroplasticity

Years ago neuroscientists made a most remarkable discovery. For decades it was thought that the number of cells in a person's brain was fixed once a child reached adolescence. From this point on the number of brain cells could only decrease. We now know this NOT to be the case. While it's been documented that chronic stress can decrease the number of brain cells (causing brain atrophy), other positive cognitive behaviors cannot only increase brain cells, but also reshape the brain. Neuroplasticity refers to the brain's ability to restructure itself after periods of training or practice (e.g., learning a foreign language, learning to play an instrument or learning to meditate). The neurological pathways can change based on a repeated experience (analogous to a dirt road becoming a highway). In the words of neuroscience, "neurons that fire together, wire together."

The Benefits of Meditation

The practice of meditation in the United States became quite popular several decades ago, first through the cultural influence of the Beatles and then under the influence of Harvard physician, Herbert Benson. Benson adapted the technique of Transcendental Meditation into a simple formula called *The Relaxation Response.* He and many people intrigued by mind-body science also conducted several research studies to determine the physiological and psychological benefits of meditation. In the past ten years, these same types of studies have investigated the benefits of mindfulness meditation. Perhaps as no surprise, both types offer the same benefits. Here are the highlights:

1 Meditation promotes better quality sleep

2 Meditation enhances the immune system

3 Meditation lowers resting heart rate

4 Meditation lowers resting blood pressure

5 Meditation increases concentration skills

6 Meditation decreases anxiety

7 Meditation increases general well-being

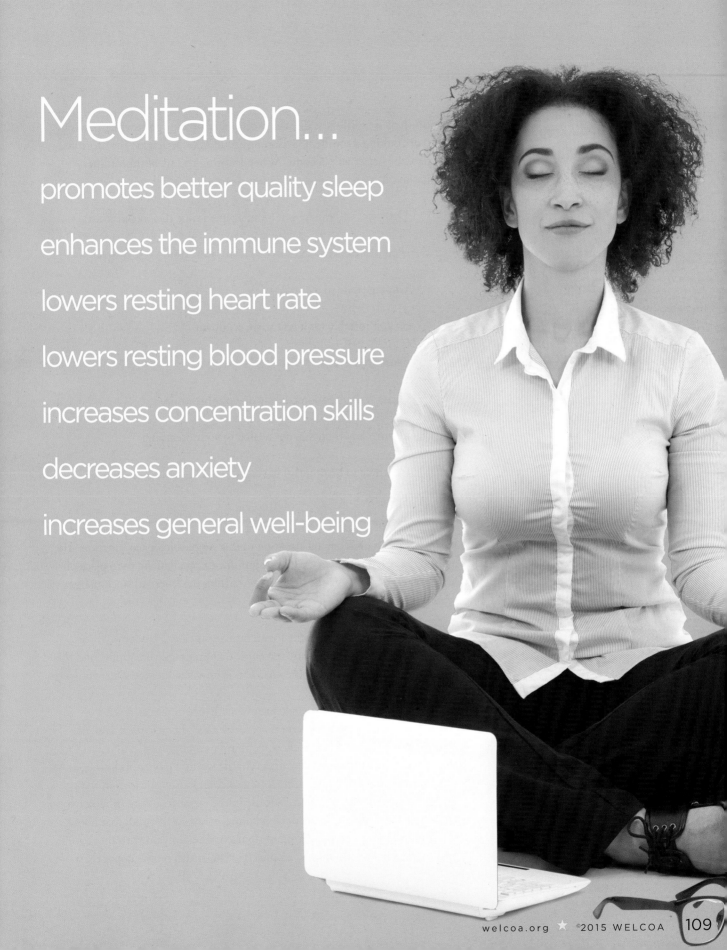

Meditation...

promotes better quality sleep

enhances the immune system

lowers resting heart rate

lowers resting blood pressure

increases concentration skills

decreases anxiety

increases general well-being

The Practice of Mindfulness

Mindfulness is a skill, just like the precise skill of your golf swing, playing piano or cooking a soufflé. Developing a skill takes practice. The more you practice, the better you become. When learning the art of mindfulness meditation, it is often suggested to start by doing the following:

1 Dedicate 5-10 minutes of uninterrupted time (before breakfast)

2 Find a quiet dedicated space to relax (away from noisy distractions)

3 Unplug from all technology

4 Sit comfortably (or if you wish, lay down)

5 Close your eyes

6 Focus your attention entirely on your breathing

7 Dismiss any thoughts not related to your breathing

8 Continue to be mindful of your relaxed breathing

The Art of Diaphragmatic Breathing

Breathing comes quite naturally to most everyone. With rare exception, we breathe without even paying attention to this simple biological function. The autonomic nervous system maintains our breathing allowing us to place our attention elsewhere (e.g., reading a book, surfing the Internet, stock market reports, etc.).

The most natural way to breathe for all humans is called "abdominal" or "belly breathing." It also goes by the name diaphragmatic breathing, and this is THE most relaxing way to breathe. This is how you breathe when you sleep.

In the western culture, few people breathe with an emphasis on their abdominal area. Instead, westerners are known as "thoracic breathers" (we tend to breath with our upper chest, not our lower abdomen). All babies are abdominal or diaphragmatic breathers. In the western culture as kids become adults, the focus of their breathing (often unconsciously) shifts from the stomach area to the upper chest, because in the western culture (whether you are a man or a woman) the media (and our egos) make us think that it looks better to have a big chest and a small stomach. The problem with thoracic breathing is that by placing the emphasis of the breath on the upper chest, we

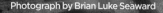
Photograph by Brian Luke Seaward

tend to also place pressure on the chest bone. Right underneath the chest bone is the solar plexus nerve bundle. When this receives pressure, a message is sent to the brain to increase heart rate, blood pressure, and many other metabolic activities that are used for fight or flight. When we redirect the emphasis from the upper chest to the lower stomach area the body begins to relax.

Placing all of your attention on your breathing is one of the hallmarks of learning mindfulness meditation. Once you can learn the simple mechanics of diaphragmatic breathing in a nice quiet space, you can take this skill anywhere.

Stages of the Breath Cycle

When you begin to focus on your breathing you may notice that there are four distinct phases of each breath cycle.

Phase 1   Inhalation (in-breath, or inspiration)

Phase 2   Slight pause (before you exhale)

Phase 3   Exhalation (out-breath or expiration)

Phase 4   Slight pause (before you inhale)

When you practice mindfulness, observe your breathing and take note of each of these four phases.

Normal Breathing

In the course of a normal day, people tend to breathe about 14-16 breath cycles a minute. This is considered normal breathing. It is interesting to note that this is about the same number of times waves hit the shore in normal weather. When people are stressed, the number of breath cycles increases, and breathing becomes more shallow. Under stress, some people can increase their breath cycles to 30 times per minute.

Mindfulness and the Art of Living in the Moment

When people describe mindfulness, they often describe it as living in the present moment. If you were to eavesdrop on the thoughts of people who are stressed, more often than not they are consumed by events in the past (often accompanied by feelings of frustration, anger and guilt), or things that might happen in the future (often accompanied by massive amounts of worrying.) Mindfulness invites you to live in the present moment by focusing on what is directly in front of you.

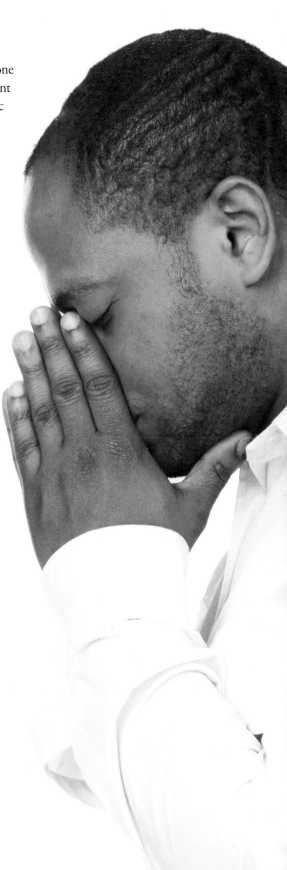

Your mind is like the sky. Clouds in the sky represent your thoughts. You look up at the sky and watch the clouds move across the sky from left to right, observing your thoughts... without judgment, without emotional attachment.

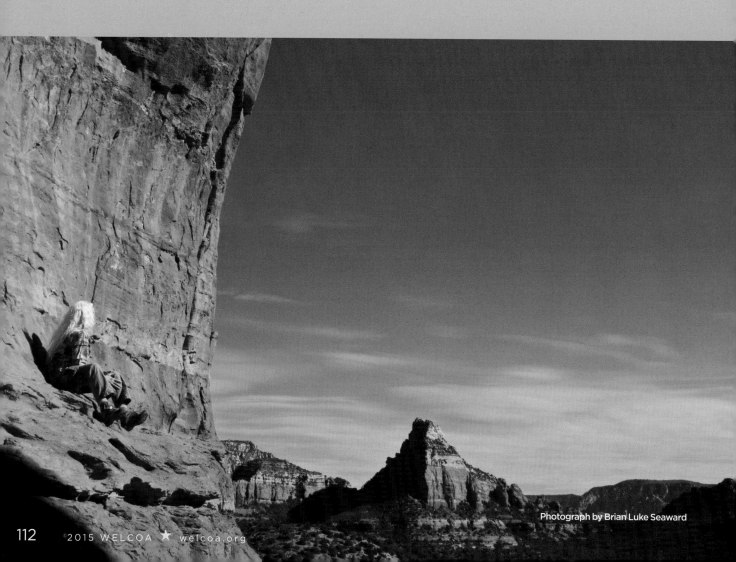

Photograph by Brian Luke Seaward

Metaphors of the Mind

Because the mind is so abstract, we often use metaphors to describe the mind. Here are two common metaphors adapted to the practice of mindfulness:

The River. Your mind is like a river; the proverbial stream of conscious thoughts. Things that float down the river (e.g., twigs, leaves, logs,) represent specific thoughts that beg for your attention. You sit on the bank of this river and observe your thoughts, watching the river flow from left to right. In doing so, you observe your thoughts without judgment, without emotional attachment.

The Sky. Your mind is like the sky. Clouds in the sky represent your thoughts. You look up at the sky and watch the clouds move across the sky from left to right, observing your thoughts… without judgment, without emotional attachment. You observe them until they fade from sight and direct your attention to the next cloud (the next issue) that begs for attention.

Mindfulness and the Art of Non-Judgment

One of the great attributes of mindfulness is to observe your thoughts without judgment; more specifically, to observe your thoughts without emotional attachment. So, to revisit the metaphor of the mind as a river, you not only observe the river of thoughts going through your mind, you take one step back and observe yourself, observing the river. When you can do this, you are truly being mindful.

Mindfulness and the Art of Domesticating the Ego

In the eastern culture, where the practice of mindfulness is mentioned, quite often the subject of ego comes up. Keep in mind that the ego is not bad. The ego, like a bodyguard that protects you from harm, is what triggers the fight or flight response when physical danger is near. For this reason, the ego is necessary. Quite often, however, the ego remains hypervigilant, reacting to things that are non-physical threats (and often to things that later turn out not to be a threat at all). In doing so, the mind becomes hijacked by the ego, and stress ensues. Mystics and sages remind us to "domesticate" our ego. By keeping the ego as bodyguard (and not CEO), we unplug from unnecessary distractions and can live in the present moment. Mindfulness meditation is a discipline to domesticate the ego so we don't have emotional poop all over the place.

> One of the great attributes of mindfulness is to observe your thoughts without judgment; more specifically, to observe your thoughts without emotional attachment.

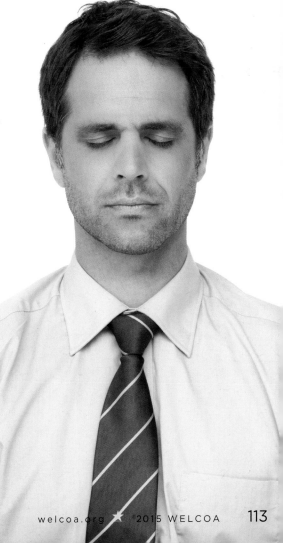

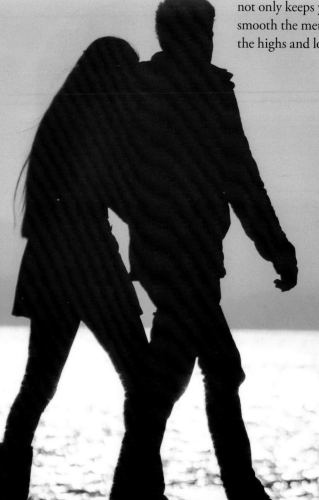

Wisdom keepers the world over have advocated the practice of mindfulness as the skill of choice to rise and walk gracefully in the midst of stress.

Mindfulness Breathing to Mindfulness Living

When Olympic athletes learn a skill, they often learn it in a quiet, non-competitive environment. Once the skill has been practiced time and time again, so that it becomes "second nature," the skill is introduced into the game of competition where it is tested and refined. The concept of transference mindfulness living can be applied the same way; from a quiet space, unplugged from distractions and the frenetic pace of life to the busy world where you live and work. This is where mindfulness will serve you best. And as we all know, a mindful way of life in the awake state will also promote a good night's sleep.

Mindfulness: A Resiliency Skill for the High-Tech Age

Resiliency is often described as the ability to bounce back after being knocked down. Chronic stress can certainly knock us down. The ability to rise gracefully after a tumble is a well-rehearsed skill. Wisdom keepers the world over have advocated the practice of mindfulness as the skill of choice to rise and walk gracefully in the midst of stress. Meditation, of any kind, not only keeps you grounded (i.e., less likely to be knocked over), but helps smooth the metaphorical waves so that your life doesn't drop so far between the highs and lows. ☾

[EXERCISE 7.1]

A Simple Mindfulness Breathing Exercise

The following is a step-by-step approach to mindfulness meditation. To begin:

A   Find a spot to sit comfortably.

B   Take off your watch (and shoes if you have these on).

C   Loosen any constricting clothing.

D   Remind yourself that for the next 5-10 minutes, this activity is all that you need to focus on.

1.   Close your eyes and give full attention on your breathing.

2.   Feel the air come into your nose or mouth.

3.   Allow your belly area to expand as you inhale.

4.   As you exhale out through your mouth, allow your stomach area to relax.

5.   Place all of your attention on your breathing.

6.   In your mind's eye, follow the flow of air in through your nose or mouth, then out your mouth.

7.   If your mind wanders, that is OK. Merely redirect your thoughts to your breathing.

8.   Notice that the exhalation is the most relaxing part of each breath cycle.

9.   Become aware of your breathing, placing all of your attention on each breath.

10.   Be mindful of how relaxed your body feels as you exhale.

11.   Repeat steps #2–#10 ten times.

12.   Open your eyes, become aware of your surroundings.

13.   Begin the rest of your day.

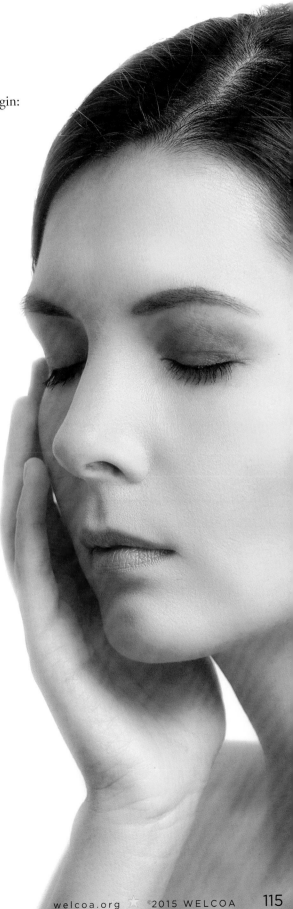

APPENDIX A

FAQ About Insomnia, Stress and Wellness

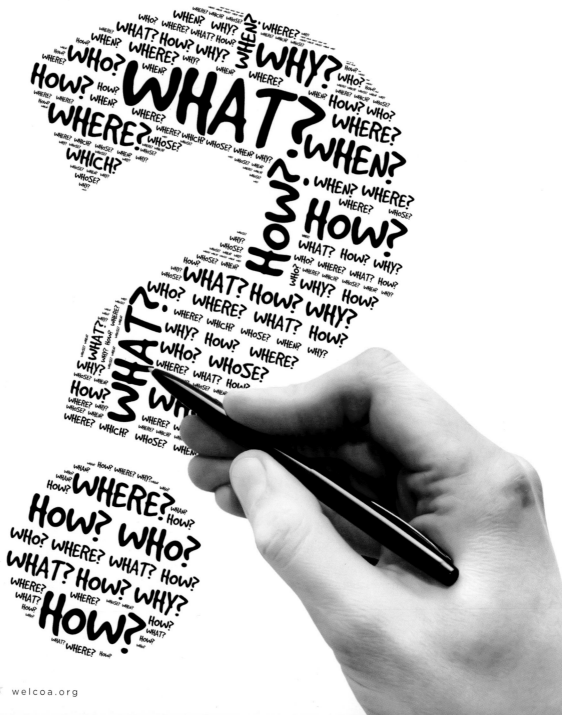

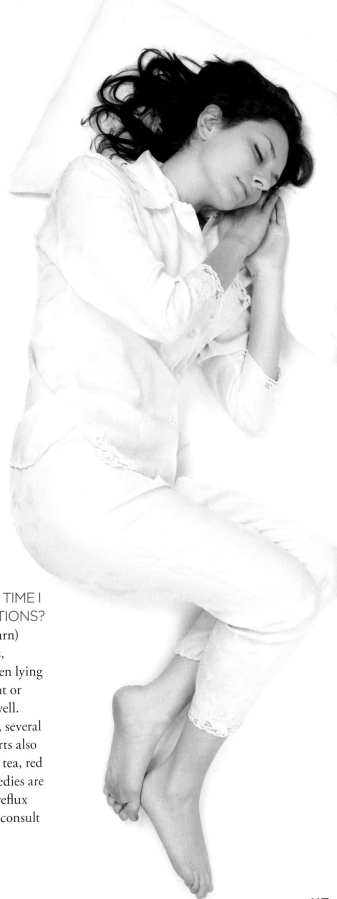

1 WHAT IS INSOMNIA?

Insomnia is often characterized as the inability to fall asleep, stay asleep or repeatedly waking up in the course of the night time hours. While some people describe insomnia as a disorder or illness, it really is a symptom of another type of health issue. The disruption of sound sleep is often suggestive of other health concerns or issues (e.g., menopause, chronic pain) or psychological problems (stress, anxiety or depression).

2 WHAT CAUSES INSOMNIA?

As described in Chapter 2, insomnia can be attributed to many factors, from the side effects of medications and menopause to restless leg syndrome and annoying house pets. Estimates suggest that psychological stress surpasses all other reasons combined as the leading cause of insomnia.

3 HOW DO I KNOW IF I AM GETTING ENOUGH SLEEP?

Research reveals that most adults need about seven to eight hours of sleep per day. Let's do the math: If you go to bed at 10:00 p.m., you would need to wake up at 6:00 a.m. Shaving off time on either end of this period may lead to fatigue in the mid morning or mid afternoon hours. Not getting enough sleep reveals itself with these characteristics; low energy, daytime sleepiness, trouble concentrating and moodiness.

4 ACID REFLUX WAKES ME AT NIGHT (THE ONLY TIME I GET IT) AND IT RUINS MY SLEEP. ANY SUGGESTIONS?

There are several reasons for acid reflux (also known as heart burn) including what is referred to as a hiatal hernia in the esophagus, allowing stomach acid to move into the throat, particularly when lying down. Acid reflux is also common in people who are overweight or obese. Smoking and drinking can aggravate this condition as well. Recommendations include eating dinner earlier in the evening, several hours before laying down and avoiding late night snacks. Experts also suggest avoiding foods associated with indigestion (e.g., coffee, tea, red meat, tomatoes, tomato sauce, garlic and onions). Natural remedies are recommended over over-the-counter pharmaceuticals for acid reflux and can be found in any health food store. If problems persist, consult your physician.

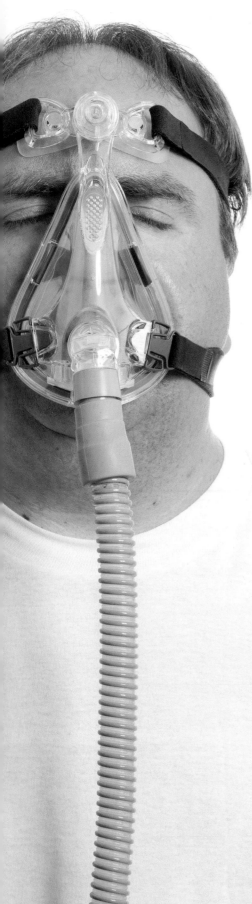

5 WHAT IS SLEEP APNEA AND HOW DOES THIS AFFECT QUALITY SLEEP?

The Mayo Clinic describes sleep apnea as a condition when breathing suddenly stops and starts. It is also described as repeated pauses in breathing. Pauses (apnea) can last for several seconds to several minutes and can occur as often as 30 times per minute. Clearly, the ramifications are serious.

One of the tell-tale signs of sleep apnea is feeling very tired after a full night's sleep and sleepiness during the daylight hours. Sleep experts note two kinds of sleep apnea. The first is called obstructive sleep apnea and occurs when the throat muscles relax to the point where the air passage is blocked. The second type is called central sleep apnea that occurs when there is some type of miscommunication between the brain and the respiratory muscles causing a cessation of breathing. Both types are very serious. Obstructive sleep apnea is more common with people who are overweight and snore loudly. Some people can have a combination of both central and obstructive sleep apnea. Most people who have sleep apnea are not aware of this condition unless a spouse or sleep partner makes them aware of it, or the individual goes to a sleep clinic and is tested.

6 CAN I CATCH UP ON SLEEP ON THE WEEKENDS?

There are two schools of thought on this topic; those of the sleep experts and those of people who engage in this activity. The experts agree that it is not really possible to catch up on your sleep. What is gone is gone. Given the fact of how much impact sleep has on our brain physiology and the immune system each night, this answer stands to reason. Even the math doesn't add up when you consider that people often shave off two to three hours a night for five or six days and then try to make this up with four to eight hours on weekends. On the other hand, people who do take an afternoon nap on Saturday or Sunday will tell you that it feels great and they wouldn't give it up for the world.

7 ARE AFTERNOON NAPS HELPFUL?

Again, there are different schools of thought on this topic. Some experts say that afternoon naps tend to throw off one's circadian rhythms and as such, will make it more difficult to get a full night's sleep. Yet, those people who take 30 minute naps in the afternoon swear by them. If you find the only way to get through the entire day is to take a short nap in the afternoon, then this may be the way to go. On the other hand, frequent afternoon naps may indicate other problems such as sleep apnea.

8 IF I CAN'T SLEEP, SHOULD I JUST START MY DAY EARLY?

Opinions may vary on this, but the general consensus is to stay in bed and leave the lights off, close your eyes and focus on diaphragmatic breathing.

Getting up and starting your day at 3:00 a.m. can create a sleep deficit, throwing off your circadian rhythms. While you may think that since you cannot sleep, you will be more productive, this is not necessarily the case.

9 CAN INSOMNIA BE LIFE-THREATENING?

Keeping in mind that insomnia is a symptom, not a disease itself, insomnia may not be life-threatening, but the cause of poor sleep may indeed be life threatening. For example, if insomnia is the result of sleep apnea, then this can be life-threatening. Insomnia may also cause a suppressed immune system which in turn, can cause a multitude of health problems, some of which are life-threatening. Once again, remember that insomnia is a symptom of a bigger problem(s).

10 IF I DON'T WANT TO TAKE SLEEP MEDICATION, IS TAKING MELATONIN A GOOD ALTERNATIVE?

Melatonin is a hormone produced in the pineal gland of the brain. It can be purchased as an over-the-counter dietary supplement used as an aid for sleeping. While taking melatonin may help to induce sleep in some people, it also signals the pineal gland not to make this hormone naturally. In turn, an outside source of melatonin can make people reliant on this type of supplement, which is not the first choice of action. Brain chemistry is very delicate. Holistically speaking, it is always recommended to address the causes of insomnia first. Finally, it is always best to check with a physician who really understands sleep disorders before experimenting on your own. Having said this, a good health care practitioner will also look to address the causes of insomnia before merely addressing the symptoms with a prescription.

11 HOW DOES ACUPUNCTURE HELP WITH INSOMNIA?

First, there are two kinds of acupuncture, Classical acupuncture and Traditional Chinese Medicine (TCM). Classical acupuncture is also known as Five-Element acupuncture. Both types work with the subtle energy of the body via the meridian pathways. Whereas TCM is primarily symptom relief based, Classical acupuncture works at the nexus of mind, body and spirit addressing both the causes and symptoms of the energy imbalance. The success rate with Classical acupuncture as a treatment for insomnia is very noteworthy.

12 AS THE PARENT OF TEENAGERS, I DON'T SLEEP UNTIL THEY RETURN HOME FROM THEIR NIGHT ACTIVITIES. ANY SUGGESTIONS?

Every parent of a teenager, particularly those who drive, has been known to lose sleep. Parenting coaches suggest that parents require teens to text or call when they arrive and depart from an event or social gathering, particularly in

Keeping in mind that insomnia is a symptom, not a disease itself, insomnia may not be life threatening, but the cause of poor sleep may indeed be life threatening.

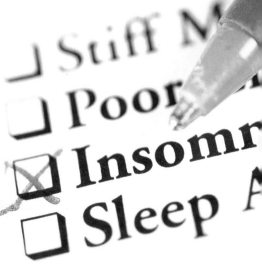

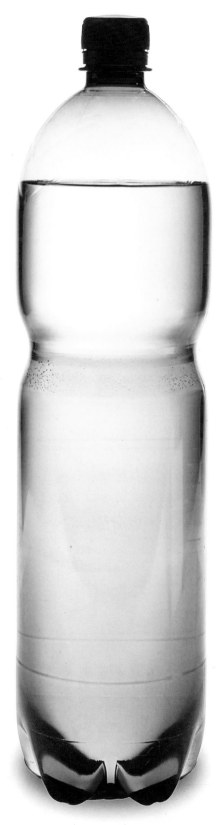

the evening. Some parenting coaches suggest that when a teen returns home in the evening that they announce their arrival to their parents (regardless of the hour) so the parents can then sleep soundly the rest of the night.

13 SHOULD I GET UP AT THE SAME TIME EVERY MORNING, EVEN ON WEEKENDS?

Chronobiology is the study of the body's internal clock, also known as circadian rhythms. Experts in the field of chronobiology suggest that even if you don't have to get up early on the weekends, your body's natural rhythms are best calibrated for health and longevity when you wake up and go to bed at the same time every day. This also includes eating meals at the same time every day.

14 WHAT IS CONSIDERED THE LATEST TIME TO DRINK FLUIDS (E.G., WATER) BEFORE BEDTIME?

Great question. Since many people wake up at night to make a trip(s) to the bathroom, disrupting a good night's sleep, one might think that drinking before going to bed is not a good idea. Yet some experts suggest having a small glass of water before bed and keeping a glass of water by your bed (they also suggest drinking some water soon after you wake up). For people who live in dry climates, this is particularly a good idea. Dehydration can also lead to fatigue. Ultimately, it becomes a matter of personal preference. It's always a good idea to empty your bladder before crawling under the covers. Perhaps equally important is developing the habit of drinking a small glass of water right when you wake up to promote good blood circulation and hydration.

15 ANY THOUGHTS ON ELECTRIC BLANKETS?

Electric blankets may be warm, even toasty, but are not recommended for your health. Please consider a down comforter. Studies investigating the effects of ELF's on the human energy field reveal that the close proximity of electrical currents to the body negatively affect one's health. For more information please read the book, *Cross Currents* by Robert Becker, MD. In his book, Becker cites a statistic in which 69% of pregnant women who use electric blankets miscarry, suggesting more than a mere coincidence. Becker also suggests to keep your alarm clock a safe distance from your head.

16 ARE SLEEPING AIDS ADDICTIVE?

Many sleeping aids contain sedating antihistamines which are known to induce sleepiness well beyond the night hours. Because they affect the delicate balance of brain chemistry, the dependence on sleeping aids may be a concern. The class of sleep medications called benzodiazepines is known to cause dependence with some people, so physicians usually advise their patients to take them for no more than a couple of weeks.

17 HOW LONG SHOULD I TAKE THE SLEEP MEDICATION?

Please ask your physician. Becoming dependent on sleep medications is never recommended. For this reason, the length of time one should take a sleep medication should be discussed before the prescription is ever written. Many people continue to use sleep medications long after they need them, thus altering the delicate brain chemistry. Remember, although medications may work to induce the desired effect of sleep, they do not address the underlying problems that often lead to insomnia.

18 IF I AM HAVING SLEEP PROBLEMS WHERE WOULD I FIND A GOOD SLEEP CENTER?

Consider looking up the American Academy of Sleep Medicine on Google. From here, you can then find an accredited center in your locale. Be sure to do your homework and ask vital questions about diagnostics and treatment as well as referrals from the clientele who have used the sleep center you intend on using.

19 DO YOU RECOMMEND EXERCISE BEFORE BED?

Exercising right before you go to sleep is not recommended. The body needs time for both an active and passive recovery after exercise. An active recovery (e.g., walking after jogging) is what is highly recommended immediately after the exercise so that the waste products can be eliminated. Sleeping right after you exercise does not allow for the body to remove metabolic waste products (e.g., lactic acid, etc.) easily. As a consequence, you may have increased muscle soreness the next morning and perhaps some other issues. Experts suggest about a two to three-hour period in between the completion of physical exercise and going to bed.

20 WHAT IS THE BEST RELAXATION TECHNIQUE TO USE WHILE TRYING TO FALL ASLEEP?

While there is no single relaxation technique that works for everyone, diaphragmatic breathing is the closet thing to a one-size-fits-all relaxation technique. Lying comfortably on your back practicing diaphragmatic breathing is one of the best ways to help induce a sound state of sleep.

APPENDIX B

Time-Tested Stress Management Tips

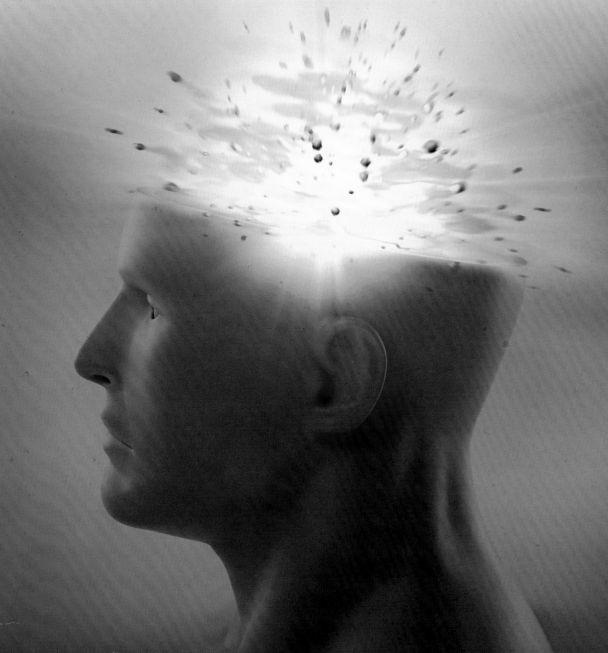

Not long ago, I was approached by a Fortune 500 Company to create a list of simple, yet effective stress management tips for their employees. Typically, I begin a talk on stress by saying this: the techniques for optimal stress management are nothing more than common sense, yet when people are stressed, common sense is not too common. This list of stress management tips is basic common sense.

Stress Tip #1
Flush The Stress Hormones Away

Walk, jog, bike, or swim each day. Exercise, in any form, is a stress to the body, but… it's "good stress" that negates the negative stress created from long traffic commutes, unending office work or common life stressors. Regular physical exercise helps reduce resting blood pressure and flushes out the stress hormones that wreak havoc on the body if/when they tend to linger for days. When you think you cannot afford the time to exercise is when you need it the most! Exercise is the next best thing to the fountain of youth!

Stress Tip #2
Reset Your Body Clock

Reset your body's clock by stepping out of the office or worksite and step into nature; a park, a riverbank, a greenhouse, a garden, even the nearest floral shop. Time spent in front of a computer—days on end—will slowly rattle your nerves on end. Recalibrate your body's rhythms to the rhythms of the natural world—every day if possible. Surround yourself in the company of trees, flowers and wildlife no matter where you live or work.

Stress Tip #3
Tense Muscle Relief

A massage, of any kind, relieves muscular tension. Muscle tension is the number one symptom of stress, whether it's sitting in traffic or in your workspace cubicle. Over time, muscle tension distorts body posture; it even compromises some organ functions. Swedish massage, Shiatsu, Rolfing, reflexology, or sports massage all have one goal; to relieve muscle tension and restore your sense of inner peace. What was once regarded as a luxury years ago is now considered a necessity in the fast-paced, information age we live in. Schedule a massage this week.

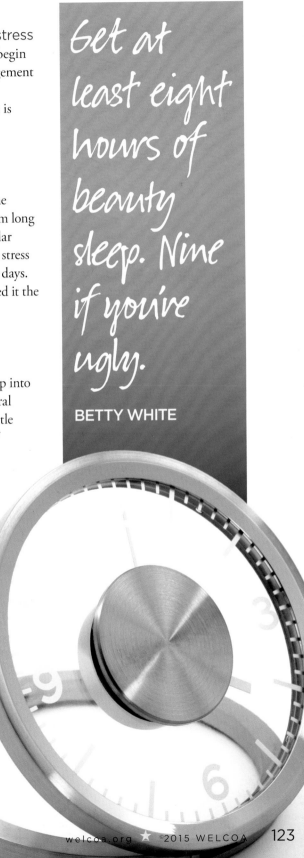

Get at least eight hours of beauty sleep. Nine if you're ugly.

BETTY WHITE

Stress Tip #4
Hydrotherapy

A hot bath, a Jacuzzi or even a long hot shower at the end of a day offers a literal and symbolic means to wash away problems. The water's heat relaxes neural endings (both skin and muscle) to induce a deep sense of relaxation to mind, body and spirit. Mineral salts and bath oils enhance the experience. Hydrotherapy is a great idea for those who have problems sleeping at night. Step into a pool of hot water tonight and let the temperature melt your problems away.

Stress Tip #5
Life Unplugged

Listening to newscasts that hype stressful national and international events for ratings only increase the stress (fight or flight) response. Repeated exposure to negativity increases blood pressure and muscle tension. During rush hour commutes as well as the dinner hour, make a habit to unplug from the hardcore newscasts that sensationalize fear. If something important occurs, trust that a friend will keep you informed and enjoy dedicated moments of silence. Briefly unplugging from all technology each day offers a respite to mind, body and spirit.

Stress Tip #6
Breathe Deep

Never underestimate the power of a good sigh. Taking a big sigh not only clears the lungs, it clears the mind (if only momentarily), of the stress at hand whether it's with traffic, staff meetings or rude people. Under duress, people tend to take short shallow breaths (or worse, hold their breath unknowingly. The latter contributes to hypertension.). Deep, abdominal breaths is the most relaxing way to breathe. Remind yourself regularly to breathe deep and enjoy the inner peace of a deep sigh.

Stress Tip #7
Establish Healthy Boundaries

Take a periodic mental health day from stress by establishing a healthy boundary between your work and your personal life. A lifestyle that is "on-demand" 24/7 is unsustainable for optimal health. Time and space away from work responsibilities often gives a fresh perspective on problems too, but you can't get this perspective without healthy boundaries. Be assertive! Create and enforce healthy boundaries in your life.

Hydrotherapy is a great idea for those who have problems sleeping at night. Step into a pool of hot water tonight and let the temperature melt your problems away.

Take a periodic mental health day from stress by establishing a healthy boundary between your work and your personal life. A lifestyle that is "on-demand" 24/7 is unsustainable for optimal health.

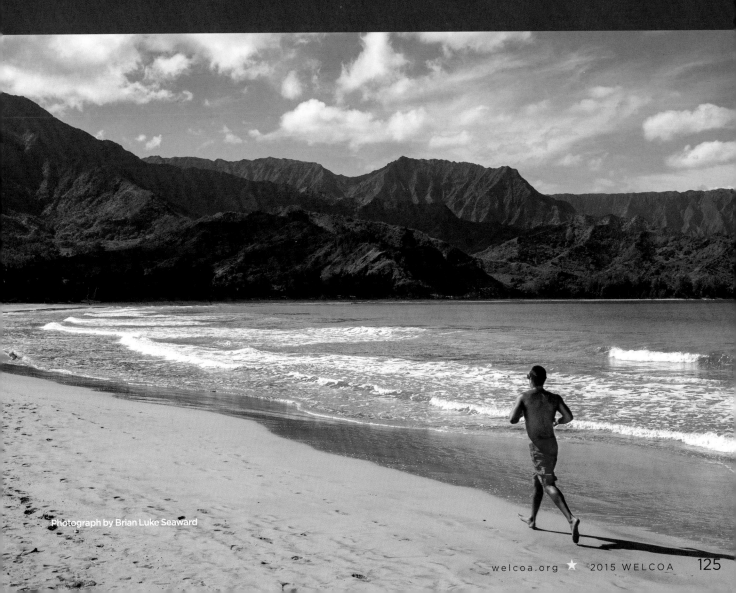

Photograph by Brian Luke Seaward

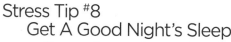

Stress Tip #8
Get A Good Night's Sleep

Down pillows and 1,000-thread count sheets are a great start to a good night's sleep but don't stop there. Remove any and all items that contribute to poor sleep hygiene... and keep a pen and pad of paper by the night stand to write down consuming thoughts that steal precious moments of quality sleep. Stress (a busy mind) is cited as the leading cause of insomnia. Minimize your stress and maximize your sleep potential. A good night's sleep boosts the immune system too!

Stress Tip #9
Furry Friends to the Rescue

Love is the greatest cure for stress and pets offer loving support in many ways. Holding a kitten, rubbing a dog's stomach or receiving a surprise kiss from a furry friend warms any heart and takes the edge off a bad day. We all need to be loved as well as express love regularly. If stress is life's toxin, than love is the antidote and house pets offer an unlimited supply of this cure.

Stress Tip #10
Tickle Your Funny Bone (Humor Therapy)

Humor heals a stressful mind. Make a point to find one funny thing to laugh at each day. Keep on the lookout for things that tickle your funny bone (e.g., jokes, photos, birthday cards, etc.). Collect them in a tickler notebook and refer to it often as your humor resource. Irony, parody, satire, blue collar, white collar or no collar; laughter is great medicine for mind, body and spirit. Remember to avoid sarcasm as it only promotes stress. Laughter is good medicine.

Stress Tip #11
Music Therapy (for the Commute)

Music, it is said, soothes the savage beast. Instrumental music (without words) soothes it best. Make a new play list of 20 soothing pieces of instrumental music that you know calms your nerves. Consider playing this relaxing musical set during long slow commutes home from work, or perhaps once you get home as a great way to unwind. Consider piano solos, Hawaiian slack-key guitar, violin concertos, Spanish flamenco and Icelandic folk music. Explore new melodies that give your mind a mini-vacation and soothe the savage beast that resides in you when tension runs high.

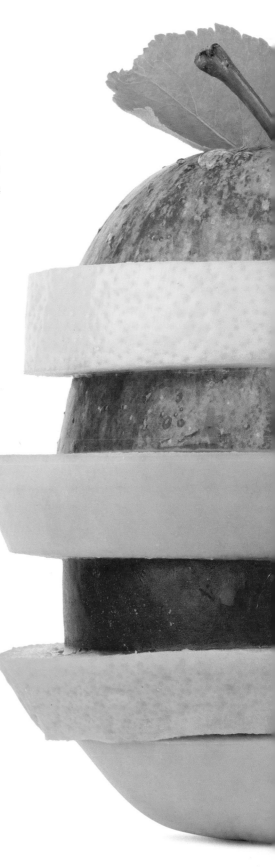

Stress Tip #12
Meditation: It's Not What You Think

Our world today is a perpetual torrent of sensory bombardment. Bits and bytes of information ricochet around our brains contributing significantly to burnout, also known as information overload. A running commentary soundtrack by one's own ego only adds to this cacophony. Meditation, known to world-class athletes as "mental training," is nothing more than a badly needed rest stop on the information super highway. It also helps increase attention span. Find a quiet place each morning, close your eyes for 5-10 minutes and think of nothing but your breathing (with long slow deep breaths). Your mind will thank you. Your body will too!

Stress Tip #13
Friends in Need

There are times to cherish solitude, and there are times to cherish good friends and family. Friends help cushion the fall of a stressful day. We don't need many friends, but we do need a handful of close friends to bond with and feel supported by in tough times. The hustle-bustle of life can often leave people with many virtual friends, but few people to call up and socialize with. Consider organizing a potluck dinner party or a small gathering of your friends and celebrate life's simple pleasures.

Stress Tip #14
Create a Relaxation Survival Kit

Stressful times call for clever measures! We take in information through our five senses. Too much information overloads the system: STRESS! We can also use the five senses to relax. Consider gathering items to soothe the body through sight, sound, taste, touch and smell (two per sense) and create a relaxation survival kit; a first aid kit for stressful times. Items in your kit might include a vile of lavender (smell), a Hawaiian Beach post card (sight), a classical CD (sound), bubble wrap (touch), and some Belgian chocolate truffles (taste). Make one for the home and office. Don't forget to replace the chocolate!

Stress Tip #15
Eat For a Healthy Immune System

Chronic stress tends to suppress the immune system through the overactive role of cortisol (the primary stress hormone). Basic living depletes essential nutrients. Chronic stress depletes them even quicker. Good quality foods can help negate the far reaches of stress to bring your immune system back into balance. Organic fruits and vegetables and free-range meats are the best sources of food to build a healthy immune system.

References & Resources

Becker, R. *Cross Currents,* Tarcher Books. New York, 1990

Davis, D., *Disconnect*. Plume Books. New York, 2011.

Dement, W. *The Promise of Sleep*. Dell Books, New York, 2000.

Ekrich, R. *At Day's Close: Night in Times Past*. W. W. Norton, New York, 2006

Glovinski, Paul. *The Insomnia Answer*. New York. Perigree Books. 2006.

Hirshkowitz M. and Smith, *Sleep Disorders for Dummies*. Wiley Publishing. New York 2004.

Krugman, Michael, *The Insomnia Solution*. New York. Warner Books. 2005.

Mass, James, *Power Sleep*. New York. Quill Books. 1999.

National Sleep Foundation (202) 347-3471 http://www.sleepfoundation.org

Park, S., *Sleep Interrupted*. Jodev Press. New York, 2012

Randall, D., Dreamland. *Adventures in the Strange Science of Sleep*. Norton Book. NY. 2012.

Turkel, S. *Alone Together,* Basic Books, New York 2012.

Resonance: Beings of Frequency: http://vimeo.com/54189727, http://topdocumentaryfilms.com/resonance-beings-frequency

Photograph by Brian Luke Seaward